THE PATH TO HEALING IS A SPIRAL

T0023042

ANNA MCKERROW

THE PATH TO HEALING IS A SPIRAL

One Woman's Journey
to Emotional Healing

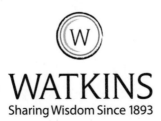

WATKINS

Sharing Wisdom Since 1893

The Path to Healing is a Spiral
Anna McKerrow

First published in the UK and USA in 2022 by
Watkins, an imprint of Watkins Media Limited
Unit 11, Shepperton House, 83–93 Shepperton Road
London N1 3DF

enquiries@watkinspublishing.com

Design and typography copyright © Watkins Media Limited 2022
Text copyright © Anna McKerrow 2022

The right of Anna McKerrow to be identified as the Author of this text
has been asserted in accordance with the Copyright, Designs and Patents
Act of 1988.

All rights reserved. No part of this book may be reproduced in any form
or by any electronic or mechanical means, including information storage
and retrieval systems, without permission in writing from the publisher,
except by a reviewer who may quote brief passages in a review.

Commissioning Editor: Ella Chappell
Assistant Editor: Brittany Willis
Head of Design: Karen Smith
Production: Uzma Taj

A CIP record for this book is available from the British Library

ISBN: 978-1-78678-615-9 (Paperback)
ISBN: 978-1-78678-629-6 (eBook)

10 9 8 7 6 5 4 3 2 1

Designed by Lapiz
Printed in United Kingdom by TJ Books

www.watkinspublishing.com

**Content warning: suicide, child illness, depression, bereavement and
explicit medical detail**

CONTENTS

"Until you make the unconscious conscious, it will direct your life and you will call it fate."

— Carl Jung

PROLOGUE

Healing is not always pretty.

When I say healing, I mean emotional and spiritual healing.

(Although, healing from surgery isn't the most gorgeous thing either, I think we can all agree – scarring, soreness, physiotherapy – but usually worth it. Plus: hospital-grade painkillers! Hurrah!)

As someone who has pursued a variety of what we might call non-traditional healing approaches for my emotional pain and mental health, I can reassure you, hand on heart, that the most effective therapies and breakthroughs I've had have been accompanied by plenty of:

- Snot
- Panda eyes
- Unattractive grunting
- Bawling

The other common feature is that usually these experiences have taken place in some remarkably underwhelming locations, including an army base, a primary school hall, various cramped suburban lounges and (my personal favourite) the room above a mechanic's workshop on an industrial estate. With the mechanic at work downstairs.

Now, I don't know about you, but I tend to imagine healing happening somewhere like a beach in Bali, where a Reiki Master called Skye rows me out to one of those houses on stilts over the crystal-clear water. As I lie face down on a treatment table, maybe listening to harp music, I watch tropical fish dart in the shallows under me and ride the waves of bliss as Skye transports me to a rainbow kingdom where I receive unimpeachable wisdom from Jesus, Ganesha and Quan Yin. Right? Surely this is what emotional or spiritual healing is all about.

Don't get me wrong, I'm saving up for Bali (and, Skye, if you're reading this, give me a call), I'm a huge fan of luxury spas and I've never met an aromatherapy massage I didn't love. Give me five-star luxury all day long please, with a side of mai tais and designer scented candles. But all I can say is that, in my experience at least, profound healing didn't come for me in a luxurious setting – which, quite honestly, is a massive bummer. I wish it had.

It came for me on drizzly days in February, where, after the session, someone's car wouldn't start and had to get towed away. It came for me in suburban semi-detached houses with grimy bathrooms, dingy south London community centres and, yes, occasionally, the odd field. I have eaten a lot of custard creams in my pursuit of better emotional and spiritual health – in fact, probably nothing symbolizes my journey to healing better than that cheapest and yet (controversially) most-loved British biscuit. I'm not complaining about the custard creams, but, you know, they're no chocolate hobnob. Don't email me with your arguments about Oreos.

Also, my healing occurred alongside, and was facilitated by, other very normal, unglamorous people. Most of the clothing choices included fleece and stretch pants. I think it's important to say this.

How do I know all this healing worked, you might ask? And why should I read your book about bawling in front of people you hardly know? How will this help me?

These are all good questions, and all I can say is that, without having participated in these healing modalities – some more effective than others, and some definitely stranger than others

– I wouldn't have been able to write this book. This is an intensely personal story, and I am not sugar-coating it for you. Some of this is hard to write, but I am writing it, because reiki, breathwork, witchcraft and communing with angels, and all the other stuff I include in this book, has enabled me to process enough of my pain to sit in front of you and bare my soul without fear. No mean feat for (actually) a very private person. So if you ask me, how do I know it worked? Well, if it hadn't, I would probably be dead about now. Seriously: there was a dark time I thought I would never get through. It also worked well enough for me to get my shit together and write this book. So, I'm alive (yay), and I'm telling you what happened in the hope that it will help you.

Why should you read this? Well, hopefully it'll make you smile here and there. Some of the things I've done in the pursuit of healing are ridiculous. I'm happy to own that.

But also, maybe, you might relate to some of it. If you've come this far, you might come a little further with me. Maybe you too have experienced loss, or illness, or held your new baby in your arms and thought, *Fuck, I'm not up to this*. Maybe you have had a seriously sick child and spent time in hospital with them. Maybe you have experienced some other terrible trauma: war, rape, miscarriage. Maybe you have grown up believing that life is all about suffering, or you find it impossible to find peace in the world as it is today. You might have experienced depression and anxiety like so many of us.

The healing modalities explained in this book may seem unglamorous or just plain odd, but for me they have offered something that mainstream solutions didn't. First, all these approaches saw me as a whole person. I wasn't a person with a wonky brain that needed fixing with some kind of magical wonder drug; I wasn't a lost cause or a burden or a weirdo. I was simply a human, having a human experience of trauma. Second, they offered me real answers about what had caused my symptoms (what you choose to believe about those answers are up to you) and, often, a real structure that explained physical, spiritual and mental health in a much more logical way than I had found elsewhere. Last, and most importantly, they worked. It's worth repeating here that, for many, drugs, cognitive behavioural therapy and traditional talking therapy also work. All I'm doing is presenting my experiences and the things that worked for me.

To return to the earlier question: how will this book help you? Well, I guess I feel that it would be a shame if you missed out on some really top-quality healing just for lack of knowledge. I'd hate to think that you might have dismissed reiki, or breathwork, or shamanic healing without fully appreciating how good it is and what it can do for you. I'd feel like I'd failed you.

In reading this book, I want you to know the nuts and bolts of the therapies – the concepts and how they work – but I also want to tell you how I, a very ordinary person, have used them. I want you to know that alternative therapies are not wishy-washy or made up, are not hugely expensive, and are definitely not only for people living in communes, wearing crystals and drinking (eating? I don't even know) kombucha. These healing techniques are for everyone. They work on everyone, in any state of mind or body, regardless of age, gender, inclination, belief or occupation.

So, imagine this book is me, a (mostly) nice, ordinary British woman in her forties that you happened to meet in the queue at the supermarket. Imagine that it's a really bloody long queue (probably Christmas) and while we're standing there, we end up having one of those weird heart-to-heart conversations that you sometimes have with strangers. I tell you about my hysterectomy and you tell me about your depression, and I say, "Hey, d'you know what really helped me with that?"

There's a saying: when you're ready, the teacher will appear. I'm going to sort of paraphrase it and say that this book is the equivalent of a random supermarket chat about reiki or conversation with someone at work about their experience with BodyTalk. It's the first-person account that can so often help us to try something new, the way that hearing from a real person about their real-life experience can be so much more helpful than reading an instruction manual.

I'm someone who has always believed in there being more to the world than meets the eye. I was brought up to be open to ideas like life after death, reincarnation and the spirit world. So maybe that meant that I wasn't as resistant to alternative healing techniques as some might be. Nowadays I'm a Reiki Master and I've found my belief system best expressed by a pagan world view (that all nature is sacred, and that there are many gods and goddesses I can connect to), as well as that of modern witchcraft, which teaches us that we can be active agents in our own growth by recognizing the subtle energies that exist in the world.

However, I'm also a mum, I have a normal job, I spend what seems like endless hours every week vacuuming and loading and unloading the dishwasher, and I spend most of my time doing normal things like binge-watching detective TV series, food shopping, cycling around rainy parks and gossiping with my friends. So, yes, by having some alternative world views to start with, I might have had fewer mental obstacles in my way when starting my healing path than some. But if that makes me a more experienced healer friend for you, then that's a good thing, right?

Whoever you are, if you've never thought about where healing could take you, let me at least show you where it's taken me. What have you got to lose?

CHAPTER 1

WELCOME TO THE WORLD OF PAIN

When I was a child, we didn't have much money. So little money, in fact, that one of the many things I have sought to heal in my adult life is what we now call "poverty consciousness", which is a phrase that I take to mean a kind of constant obsession with and fear of being poor. Poverty consciousness means that you always feel poor, no matter how much money you actually have. It also means that when you have money you tend to instantly self-sabotage yourself by spending it as quickly as humanly possible, because you feel wrong or uncomfortable having it, thereby putting yourself back in the more familiar position of wanting it but not having it. It's not that you consciously enjoy the lack – in fact, you hate it. But you still can't stop fixating on money, rather than having a relaxed and healthy attitude toward it.

Sound familiar? It sure does to me! I have spent a long time healing my way out of that one. Poverty consciousness is endemic in society. (I could write a whole other book about it.) The point that I am circling here is that I am not writing this book from a place of wealth or from a history of one. Most of the therapies and experiences I talk about can be found at low cost, or researched more in books from the library and on YouTube. Your journey to better emotional and mental health need not cost you more than you have, but at the same time, it is worth every penny and every hour you spend on it.

Conversely, I've also found that the more healing I did, the better relationship I had with money. Money is, in fact, intensely emotional. We can desire it and feel like we never have enough. Global stock markets rise and fall on subjective popularities, unpopularities, predictions and other unscientific impulses. We fear money will corrupt us. It has been described as "the root of all evil". Money gets a rough deal, all in all.

I was an only child and grew up with my mum, a single parent. My parents got divorced when I was about two, and I saw my dad every other Saturday from about eleven o'clock in the morning to five in the afternoon (he lived in another city about two hours away from us, and, after a couple of years, met his second wife). He would take me out for the day, providing the fast-food lunch that my mum couldn't afford and would never buy. Can anything beat fried chicken followed by an individual trifle? Even today, I buy myself packs of ready-made trifles with glee from the supermarket.

As a parent now, I realize how wise they were to separate when I was that young and I'm grateful for it, but for a long time I wasn't. As an adult, I can be realistic about the fact that, quite often, people don't find their true loves until later in life, or not at all. I also realize now that marriage is hard and, often, it doesn't work – and there's no shame in separating if it's better for the children and for you. A happier single parent is way better than a miserable marriage. But, when I was a kid, I wanted my dad.

Dad seemed the most fun person in the world. When he visited, my mum described to me, it was like he turned a special light on for me so that everything was bright and wonderful. He still does that now, and I love him for it. He is hilarious, silly, kind, generous, philosophical about the world, humanitarian, a great musician, charming and welcoming to strangers. But he is also human. He has off days, as we all do. As a kid, I wasn't around to see the off days and so he was perfect in my eyes. Mum went on to explain that, because she was there all the time, she couldn't have her light on as bright as that every day or it would burn out. No one could. So if she seemed not as bright, not as fun, not as hilarious or willing to buy fried chicken for lunch and take me to the zoo, then it was because she was working hard to support us and put food on the table every day.

I remember that conversation so well, because it came about when I guiltily confessed to her that I'd told a friend that I loved Daddy more than Mummy. Afterwards, I was racked with guilt. I knew it wasn't true, and I knew that, if anything, I had a deep, almost terrifying love for her that came from our intense one-to-one relationship. Sure, Dad was fun, but Mum did everything. She was everything and everyone to me: wise counsellor, teacher, chef, patient explainer, fixer of broken taps, disciplinarian, play-date host, birthday-cake maker, and everything else. She was the person who explained what life was all about, who weathered my tantrums, who listened to my teenage troubles, told me about sex (with the help of a book she'd borrowed from the library – she was thorough and made a point of being marvellously unembarrassed about the whole thing), made my school skirts and carried me home from the doctor in her arms when I was ill.

Outwardly, I was philosophical about not having Dad around, but, secretly, I envied other families that did have dads. I'd watch them, wide-eyed, at the dinner table when I went to friends' houses for play dates after school and marvel at their loud voices and how everyone seemed to wait for their opinions. I wondered why they got bigger dinners than everyone else – in our house, I got the biggest bowl of Angel Delight and the most roast potatoes. Yet, in retrospect, I don't remember those dads in much detail or how they interacted with their children – on the rare occasions they did, in many cases – and sometimes I was shocked at how dull they were. It was more that they were just *there*, and I wished my brilliant, bright Dad could be there at the dinner table with us. I would even have given up a roast potato or two.

Mum took the divorce hard. It was her decision, which tells you everything you need to know about her: she wasn't afraid of doing difficult things, even when they broke her heart. She knew it was right that her and Dad divorce, even in the late 1970s when divorce carried far more stigma than it does now, and being a single mother was worse. When I was older, she told me about all the times that neighbours' husbands sneaked around to our house, propositioning her – and the time when the family doctor told her to come and sit on his knee and describe what was wrong with her. Being a divorced – and attractive – woman in the 80s was not an easy ride. It took time for other women to trust her, trust that she wasn't going to run away with their husbands. (Which, remembering the choice in our neighbourhood at the time, was laughable.) It meant that those early years were lonely for her.

She was heartbroken. She was such a pure, naïve and loving young woman that the idea of not being married and sailing into the sunset with a happy family was unthinkable. Like so many of her generation, her own parents' marriage hadn't been perfect (reading between the lines as an adult now, my grandmother should also have left my grandfather, but it just wasn't done then – and wasn't possible with five children and no job) but she'd thought that was normal; she'd thought that family life was still the ideal for a woman. She should have had other children; she should have had a loving husband and a home that she could have made beautiful. It was all she wanted. I still feel that sadness for her; she didn't deserve what happened. Yet we all experience pain at some time or another. I personally believe that pain is part of the human condition (what a cheery world view! But I mean it in a positive, inclusive kind of way. Ha!) and it's our responsibility to heal and transmute it somehow. When I did some shamanic training, my teacher Simon talked about this material world as the *world of pain*. Not like in the phrase, "If you do that you'll be in a world of pain" or whatever. Like, a literal world of pain. Here on Earth, pain is what we souls have come here to experience, along with love and all the rest of the human experience.

4

But why would our souls choose pain – physical, emotional, mental? Surely it's to be avoided at all costs? It's a bit of a counter-intuitive concept, especially if you've been raised in a largely secular society informed by a Judeo–Christian world view (as I have). If you are a Hindu or a Buddhist, you have a different view of how pain and destruction feature in life. In Hinduism, you have the goddess Kali whose purpose on Earth is destruction. She is the ending of all things. She is the pain that comes so that the healing may begin. She is the dark so that the dawn may break. Kali is to be honoured, like any other god, as having her natural space in the universe.

Alternatively, Buddha teaches us about the "two arrows". The first arrow is pain, which is inevitable. The second arrow is when we "shoot" ourselves with fear, resistance and judgement of the pain. If you are a Buddhist, you are taught to have a relationship with pain rather than ignoring it, medicating it away and denying it ever exists. Physically (and mentally and emotionally), pain exists to tell the body/mind/heart that something is wrong. Pain is a symptom. It is not the original problem.

Living in Judeo–Christian-influenced cultures means that we are more likely to have a strictly binary view of the world: good–bad, light–dark, heaven–hell, pain–pleasure, male–female. In the Christian view, we must strive toward goodness; heaven is the goal in the afterlife and we are supposed to resist the devil on Earth who plagues us with pain, suffering, sex, "temptation" and human frailty.

For me, it makes a whole lot more sense to consider our lives on this material plane of Earth as a place where we learn to live with pain and to heal from it. If Earth is as generous as it is in providing countless opportunities for suffering, there must be a reason. I see pain as part of being human, and in our pain we have opportunities to heal and become powerful beings.

There is no real reason to attach emotional judgements to pain or to things like disease. It's hard not to, of course. We're terrified of diseases because they cause pain, discomfort and sometimes death, but viruses and bacteria and other things like cancers and inherited conditions are not inherently evil. All we can really say about them is: they exist. We can mitigate against them by cleanliness, vaccination, medication and maintaining healthy lifestyles, but they're part of our lives. Pain in itself is not evil. There's no consciousness to it; it's just your mind/body/heart saying, *I need help*. So, in many ways, pain is a good thing if it signposts us to help ourselves.

As for the rest of the suffering in the world? Humans created it all, because humans are imperfect beings. All we can do is accept it, decide how best to respond to it in a responsible and caring way and, I believe, raise our own personal "vibration" by doing our own healing work. When we heal ourselves, we can then make choices that don't perpetuate the existing patterns that we find repellent in the world (I think it's important to phrase it this way, because there are many truths and beliefs in the world, and as long as they come from a place of love and compassion, how can any of them be wrong?). For example, you do some healing and feel strong enough to come out as a lesbian, thereby living your own life more authentically and helping to move humanity forward toward greater LGBTQ+ visibility and acceptance. Or I do some healing around my trauma about being bullied and then feel able to end my abusive relationship, indicating to my partner that that behaviour is not acceptable. Our healing enables us to act.

Like many people, my mum never gave herself an opportunity to heal. She held on to that pain without asking for help, and I grew up feeling her depression and pain, even though she tried to hide it. She thought she was protecting me. That's what we all do for our kids, right? We plaster on a smile and we get on with life. But they know. Trust me, they always know.

That experience of living with her pain was what broke my heart. Not so much my dad not being there, which was regrettable but okay. It also led me to the healing she would never allow herself to have. In a way, she showed me the blueprint of pain, and when I was much older I became determined not to repeat what I thought of as her mistakes. She did not heal, so she could not act. I chose to heal, and one of my actions is to share this story with you, hoping that it will help in your healing.

If we believe that pain is an acceptable and inevitable part of life, then we can't ever judge anyone for making "mistakes" – after all, to err is human. Mum simply lived her life in the way that she chose to. It was her life and her journey, and if healing (and generally living life) has taught me anything over the years, it's that we are all on our own journey, and it's pointless to judge others. Walk a mile in someone else's shoes, as the saying goes. In my view, everyone is here on Earth to experience something, but it's not a set curriculum. One size does not fit all. All I can tell is my story.

When my mum was diagnosed with cancer when I was twenty, I was furious with her. This is a common experience, I think, when someone we love falls critically ill or is threatened in some way. Much in the same way as when your kid falls over after jumping off the wall when you've just said, quite clearly, "Don't jump off that wall", and starts crying, your initial reaction is to shout at them, before you quickly move to concern and checking for broken bones. It's the same emotional response. I was furious at Mum for having cancer because I felt that I'd already lived with her pain all these years, which I HATED – why couldn't she move on? Be happy? – and now I had to cope with her cancer. She was involving me in her suffering once again.

Now, I know that this response is not kind. It is not caring. And yet, my mum was the most kind, caring person when it came to other people's suffering. People used to flock to her and tell her their problems as if she was a pain magnet – in the shopping centre, in the dentist's waiting room, on the bus (highly embarrassing to me as a teenager). *Come to me, your moany and your groany*, I'd think. I'd have been harangued into going to the supermarket with her when I really wanted to be at home reading, and then I had to wait while some woman offloaded all her problems and Mum just stood there and took it.

I hated it. My mum had what I would now describe as no healthy boundaries when it came to other people's pain. She was a psychic sponge. She took it all in. The other woman (always a woman; men didn't talk to her in public – she was the Divorced Woman after all, and likely a succubus) would skip away after half an hour or so of pouring out all her troubles, and my mum would figuratively hoist them onto her back and get on with the shopping.

Nowadays, I know that psychic defence is very important. I take salt baths; I try to remember to do a daily grounding meditation; and I invoke archangels to protect me from other people unconsciously dumping their emotional sludge into my energy system. No, thank you! Plus, you know, I have resting bitch face and am gifted with a natural *fuck off* vibe.

But Mum did not know or have any of those things, and, as a natural psychic and empath, people would run to her side, ready to vomit their shadowy emotions at her. So I was already instinctively angry at her for not having boundaries, something I felt but couldn't verbalize for a long time until I realized what was happening. And then, on top of that, now she was ill.

When people are seriously ill, other people will try to reassure them and you, the family member, that everything is okay and will be okay. Yet, it is not okay. Sometimes, illness never gets better. And even if it does, it can be a hugely traumatic experience.

I remember one night having a very vivid dream. (I'm generally a vivid dreamer, always have been. In fact, as a heads up, there will be lots of dreams described in this book.) In the dream, my mum had a large hole through one of her feet. A family friend was with me, looking at it and telling me, "It's okay, it's nothing, don't worry, it's not a big deal." And in the dream I was so angry at that person because it *was* a big deal. My mum had a hole all the way through her foot! How could she walk? Why was everyone saying it was okay?

I was furious on waking up from that dream because I was furious with all the people around me who, out of kindness, were trying to minimize the impact of Mum's cancer for me. But I wanted someone to acknowledge how shitty it all was. I wanted to cry and be sad, which is a normal reaction when a loved one is diagnosed with a possibly fatal condition. By smiling it all away, the people around me made me feel that I was wrong for being negative. And that made me angry and resentful. I was *so angry*!

I knew, rationally, that it wasn't Mum's fault she was ill. But I felt that she had somehow wished it upon herself. I felt, somehow, that all the emotional gunk she'd let other people dump on her all those years had built up into a cancerous mound inside her. And it seemed to me that all the pain and trauma she had insisted on hanging on to from the divorce had metastasized into the lump that was now threatening my wellbeing and hers.

Here, I would like to stop briefly and clarify that I do not believe that when people are ill, they have brought it on themselves, or consciously/unconsciously wished it to happen in some way. One sees this simplistic, victim-blaming train of thought a lot in New Age circles and I want to address it here before we go on.

Being human means that we are vulnerable to disease, whether that is inherited, a genetic predisposition or a viral or bacterial infection. We are also vulnerable to accidents and mental health issues. Having a good immune system is a brilliant thing, but your immune system cannot protect you from diseases such as polio, Covid-19, cancer, yellow fever and AIDS.

Cancer Research UK now says that one in two people will experience cancer in their lifetime, which immediately puts the "you make it happen" idea in the "unlikely" category. More and more, cancer is just something that happens now.

You can for sure avoid doing some things that may increase your likelihood of becoming ill: you can stop smoking, make sure you exercise, eat vegetables, drink water and avoid becoming an alcoholic. Other than the obvious things, there are no ways to prove that anyone has made any illnesses or conditions appear in themselves, and certainly not from "being negative". I do think it's true that people can hold on to trauma, and that can affect them as time goes on.

However, my mum did not want to die from cancer. Nobody wants cancer.

When we'd gone to the hospital for the result of her mammogram that time, we had made a day of it. We were going to pop in and get the routine results, then go shopping and have lunch. We'd already been to a homeware shop on the way and bought some new wine glasses. Mum hardly ever took a day off work – including weekends – so it was a real occasion.

As we sat opposite the doctor, who, gently, told us that the results of the mammogram showed "some abnormalities", I learned something else I hadn't known about Mum – that she'd had an abortion when I was about eight or nine. She'd never mentioned it, even now that I was twenty and grown up enough to understand.

In retrospect, knowing that made so much sense in understanding Mum's ongoing pain. All that time, I'd thought it was just the divorce. *Why couldn't she get over it and move on?* I'd always ask myself, rationalizing that people got divorced all the time. Now, I understood a little more. She was a single, divorced mother, living on the breadline, who'd accidentally got pregnant from her then-boyfriend and, I'm guessing, didn't feel able to cope with another baby. She would have been around forty then.

I don't know what her abortion experience was like. I suspect that it wasn't all that good. This was around 1986 or 1987, and I can hazard a guess that even qualifying for an abortion at that time would have been difficult as an unmarried woman, never mind the actual experience.

I don't know whether she talked about it with friends afterwards. She didn't want to talk about it with me once I found out, apart from the basic details, and we never spoke about it again after that day. I regret that, but I didn't know how to bring it up, and she could be pretty stubborn when she wanted to be.

There is research now that suggests the trauma of abortion can cause post-abortion stress syndrome (PASS), a kind of PTSD. Symptoms include guilt, anxiety, numbness, flashbacks to the surgery itself (usually conducted while you are awake) and suicidal thoughts. This isn't to say that most women who have an abortion experience these things; for many women it's a positive thing, and PASS should never be used as an anti-abortion argument. Abortions are needed for all sorts of reasons, and it is good that counselling now exists for those that want it afterwards. I've had a hysterectomy (more on this later!) and for me, it was nothing less than completely joyful: a relief and a new lease of life. Yet for many women, the situation around a hysterectomy may be more charged with regret, trauma and fear, as well as the many physical complications that can arise. In all potentially traumatic situations, I say, people should be offered support if they want it. And being a healing advocate, of course, I would also highly recommend the "alternative" therapies I talk about in this book.

I think abortion was traumatic for Mum. She was alone, she had it in secret (I think one neighbour knew, as they had me for a sleepover overnight), she wasn't in a stable relationship for support (and was being stigmatized for that at the time) and then didn't have any counselling afterwards. I think, knowing how stoic and yet self-blaming she was, she would have felt like a bad mother and a bad woman, but she also would have thought that she didn't need help because, "Life is full of pain and it's your job to keep going and be strong." That's what she taught me, and it has taken me a long time – I'm forty-four! – to unlearn it. It isn't true. For all the fellow stoics out there, repressing your emotions and "getting on with life" – there is another way, which is the Way of Being Less Hard on Yourself. It is the Way of Giving Yourself a Break. Say it with me: "Give yourself a break." And don't forget to breathe.

It still hurts me to know that Mum didn't get any help – counselling, healing, whatever – because she didn't do anything wrong, either by being a single mum, being divorced or having an abortion. I still wish that she could have had either a strong friendship group that would have held her through those difficult, lonely years, or a loving partner who would have held her hand, drowned her in hugs and made her endless cups of tea. I hope with all my heart that she gets a life of love in her next life. In this one, she experienced a lot of trauma.

As we'll learn later, there are models of healing the energy body (reiki, for example) where the theory is that trauma makes its way into the physical body through the outer realms of the emotional and spiritual bodies – your aura, if you like. Christian Flèche says in his book *The Biogenealogy Sourcebook: Healing the Body by Resolving Traumas of the Past*[1]:

> *"Activation of illness" is the body's reaction to unresolved events that are frozen in time. These unresolved traumas affect the body on the cellular level and manifest in minor as well as more serious chronic conditions.*

In my experience and in my observations of others, I can see that Flèche (and many others who take this view) has a point.

Mum beat the first round of cancer. It was breast cancer; she had a mastectomy. She was given radiotherapy and tamoxifen, and it worked. It went away, or appeared to, and a shadow lifted from our lives. Yet I was still very angry, though I pushed it deep down inside myself.

That shadow lifted for almost ten years, but a month after my thirtieth birthday, Mum was dead.

---

[1]   Healing Arts Press, 2008

CHAPTER 2

CRYING WITH STRANGERS IN COMMUNITY CENTRES

As I received my reiki one attunement, I started to bawl.

I was in a room full of people who had been complete strangers until the night before when I'd rocked up to a residential centre – no doubt more commonly used for school trips and scout activities – and taken part in a very awkward "getting to know you" drinks where everyone drank tea and made shy comments about the weather. I tried to control my natural impulse to find someone in the group to make inappropriate jokes with; this was after all a very serious HEALING WEEKEND.

What was going on in my life at this point? It was three years before Mum died, and I was living in London, sharing a flat with my boyfriend of the time and generally having fun in the way one should do in their twenties: parties, drinks after work and meals out we couldn't really afford. (In fact, I was working up a pretty impressive pile of debt I'd have to deal with a couple of years later.)

However, I had been feeling more and more dissatisfied with *just* going to work in the day and getting drunk in the evenings; I knew I needed something more in my life. I had found my reiki teacher giving out free reiki sessions at my local community centre, and I knew afterwards that it was something I wanted to pursue. Reiki filled a sense of yearning I had for more meaning, more spiritual connection to something outside myself.

Reiki is a Japanese healing technique, formulated by a guy called Dr Mikao Usui in the mid-19th century. Dr Usui, a Buddhist, had trained in a variety of healing and meditation practices before discovering the reiki symbols after 21 days of fasting and meditation up a mountain. The symbols he discovered are the ones we use today – Japanese symbols that, when drawn with the hand and channelled into a human energy body, transmit four slightly different healing energies into the receiving person's energy field. You become able to give reiki to other people, and to work with the energy yourself, when you have what's called an attunement. There are three levels of attunement in reiki.

With reiki one, you are attuned to reiki energy (in a way, you're tuned in like a radio to the right wavelength) and you learn how to heal yourself and others with the hands-on techniques. With reiki two, you are given two of the four reiki symbols that provide you with more specific ways to heal on physical and emotional levels, and also one multidimensional symbol that enables you to heal outside of time and space limitations. This means you can send reiki to people you aren't physically present with, and you can also send healing backward and forwards in time. Truly fifth-dimensional shizzle right there.

The final reiki level is Reiki Master, where the Master symbol is given to you in your attunement. The Reiki Master symbol name translates in English as "bright shining light" or "great enlightenment" from Japanese. I'll touch on what Master level is like later, but for now, believe me when I say it's kind of like connecting to the secret matrix of the universe (oh, is that all?), and adds an extra oomph to your healing work.

The symbols themselves are the same for everyone: it's genuinely a one-size-fits-all arrangement. They're drawn/channelled/transmitted into your energy body by a Reiki Master when you have an attunement – which, in practice, means that you sit quietly, probably listening to some nice music, and the Reiki Master stands behind you and draws the symbols above your head. For them, it's a more complex meditative experience involving certain breathing techniques, visualizations and mantras. When the symbols are "in", you're done. You let them bed in for about a month, but essentially that's it, and though you call on them and say their names when you give a reiki treatment to yourself or someone else, the reiki is basically always "on" from then onwards: it's not something you can really turn "off". It's more that it just becomes a part of you. This isn't at all alarming, by the way. It's not tiring, and you don't suddenly enter a strangely enchanted life full of mermaids and the like (well, I haven't, anyway). It's just that you're now connected to a universal healing ray, and it works through you, and in you, at all times.

The rest of the time you spend with a reiki group or teacher will involve learning about how the energy body works, including the chakra system. Some teachers will go into other areas, like using crystals, or you might have a teacher who is also into yoga or a Buddhist, and so some of those things can be learnt and combined into your reiki practice. Fundamentally, the most important part of using reiki is the symbols. The four symbols open your psychic, emotional energy body to the high-vibrational healing current.

When you have a reiki treatment, the idea is that the practitioner channels universal energy through their hands and into the energy body of the person they are treating, helping them relax, clear their mental, emotional, physical and spiritual energy bodies of blockages and stresses and thereby helping them heal themselves. It's a minimal contact healing technique, so when you give a treatment, usually your hands hover somewhere above the person's body, though sometimes you might rest your hands gently on the body, too.

So, this is what I had signed up for on my reiki one attunement weekend. As I mentioned earlier, it was held at a rather nice residential centre and there was a significant amount of tea drinking and cake eating. After some getting-to-know-you chat, we started to learn about the energy body. In brief, this means that around your physical body there are other, less dense layers of energy that carry thought, emotions and energy. They are tethered specifically to you and also part of the greater world/universal energy matrix. The energy body also includes the energy centres, or chakras, primarily the seven most well-known ones that are the colours of the rainbow and follow the spine from the base to the crown of the head (though there are others too).

Before the attunement took place, we'd held hands and swayed to Elton John's "Tiny Dancer" – never breaking eye contact. After that we'd sung Billy Joel's "The River of Dreams". (A lyrics sheet was provided in case you didn't know the words.) What was the point of the singing, you ask? I think, in retrospect, it was about raising energy as a group and within the space we were working in. High-vibrational music and sound can be key in creating the right "feel" for many situations, as we all know. Consider watching a high-tension murder scene in your favourite crime drama with a bouncy pop soundtrack. Not scary.

The eye contact – and almost aggressive levels of smiling – was, to my mind, a little much, but I decided to put my British reserve to one side and beam back at everyone else as best I could. My approach to all healing activities has always been that I might as well get everything I can from it: I'm nothing if not an I'm-here-now-I-might-as-well person. That said, smiling and singing and holding hands with strangers felt like a cult activity in that moment, and quite frankly I think it would feel the same if I did it again now. As well as the eye contact, there was also quite a lot of friendly winking. Make of that what you will.[1]

Joking aside, though, I really noticed the energy that the people facilitating the course had created in the room.

---

[1] It definitely wasn't a cult, just to be clear. I've seen various documentaries and I know the important differences: no one revealed a secret ammunition locker, we were not required to get naked at any point, no one claimed to be the Son of God, and the strongest drug present was – you guessed it – tea.

It was *zingy*. It was sort of hot without being hot. It was a very ordinary room, but, somehow, the energy had lifted in it. The mood was giggly and a bit silly – I liked that no one was taking themselves too seriously – but also sincere and focused. This was the reiki energy at work, and the facilitators, Reiki Masters, had specifically charged the room, creating and holding this very warm, welcoming space for us. Later, I learned that this was done with methods as diverse as singing (see above), drumming, incense, crystals, tracing the four reiki symbols in the air with their hands, channelling the energy, chanting and prayer.

In fact, a piece of classical music was playing when Pennie, the Reiki Master leading the course, stood behind me and traced the reiki symbols into my aura. I burst into tears at the point when the strings held a particularly high, drawn-out note.[2] I remember saying something like, "Sorry, it's this lovely music making me cry!" She replied by telling me to breathe. Turns out, getting your reiki attunement is not widely regarded as a time to chat.

The music *was* lovely, but it wasn't just that. I felt a huge rush of energy through me, like a fire, and it pushed a knot of emotion up through my body and into my throat. Have you ever had that feeling when you're suddenly overcome by emotion? When you just can't do anything about it?

It was really strange, having it then, without a reason for it. I wasn't in the middle of an argument. Nothing sad had just happened. Yet, the process of attunement enabled this energy to move through me, and I cried. I bawled in front of the 15 or so other people in the room, without being able to stop. And it was okay. They just smiled and told me to breathe.

---

[2]   The piece of music was Jules Massenet's well-known "Thaïs, Act II: Méditation" from his opera *Thaïs*. In the first scene of Act II, Athanaël, a Cenobite monk, confronts Thaïs, a beautiful and hedonistic courtesan and devotée of Venus, and attempts to persuade her to leave her life of luxury and pleasure and find salvation through God. Perhaps (as a long-time devotee of Venus, goddess of love and luxury) this is why I cried.

In healing, music is used in a variety of ways (later, I'll talk about a breathwork session that used Eminem to great effect), both to encourage emotions to rise to the surface, and (in the case of something like a gong bath) to induce a level of theta brainwave relaxation in order to heal the body. Theta waves are a kind of neural activity that happen in REM sleep and in meditation. Being in a theta state means that you can withdraw from the conscious mind and "communicate" directly with the unconscious, which directs autonomic brain functions, memory and emotion. Some people, including me, believe that this state is a good one in which to address trauma. During a gong bath, or when you listen to a drum at a particular rhythm, or with a variety of other sound-induced methods (there are loads of lovely hours-long tracks you can find on YouTube, for example), you can enter into that self-healing zone while being awake. There are lots of great books available on the fascinating area of sound healing, some of which I've listed at the end of this book.

I once attended a gong bath session that made me so intensely furious I had to leave before the end. The next day, I told my boss about it, and she said, "Oh, gong baths make everyone furious. You're lying there trying to listen to the gong and all you can focus on is some guy in the room sniffing. STOP SNIFFING!"

In my case it was a woman called Sue with a relentless cough, but close enough. JESUS, SUE – MAYBE SEE A DOCTOR FOR THAT. I mean, I'm not one to judge (full disclosure: I really, really am), but if I had a hacking cough, I wouldn't go to a gong bath. Even in pre-pandemic times. Just saying.

I guess the point is that the gong bath worked, though, as it helped release this furious anger that I and my boss obviously had stored up, just waiting to be trapped in a lavender-scented room for an hour with a constant sniffer/cougher.[3]

Anyway, I digress. Back to the reiki attunement.

---

[3] Obviously, I would still highly recommend gong baths to anyone. Most people probably find them very relaxing; My boss and I are perhaps just naturally furious people.

After the attunement I felt pretty crappy. I spent about a week crying, on and off. *Crying?* At this point in my life, I'd been a non-crier for years. I'd schooled myself in the art of stoicism, and, if I really had to cry, I'd do it on my own, at night, in bed, silently. This was where I was with my emotions, and it wasn't a great place to be. However, I'd decided at an early age that silently crying alone in your room was the best thing for everyone because a) no one likes a wimpy crybaby, b) other people had worse problems and, most of all, c) I didn't want to worry my mum.

The thing is that when you've spent most of your life beating yourself up when you feel sad and hiding your emotions (and making yourself a bit of a martyr in the process, if I'm honest), you are angry as hell. My anger was directed at certain people (at that point I was subconsciously angry with my dad, although we continued to have a good relationship and I still adored him) but, in retrospect, I was mostly angry with myself for enacting this repressive standard of stoic emotion-squashing. I was resentful at not allowing myself to cry, at not allowing myself to receive the comfort and understanding I would give to my friends. Perhaps I knew that actually I was (and am) a *very* emotional person, and that once I opened the floodgates, I wouldn't be able to close them.

Ah, the crying. This was not what I'd signed up for! Surely I was supposed to be feeling amazing? Yet I realized, after that week of purging, that I *did* feel better, and that I'd released some of that resentment. I hadn't realized I'd been holding so much.

Turns out, we all need to cry. Regularly, in fact. Crying reduces the body's manganese level, a mineral that affects mood and is found in significantly greater concentrations in tears than in blood serum. Elevated manganese levels can be associated with anxiety, irritability and aggression. Tears also help humans eliminate stress hormones like cortisol that build up during times of emotional turmoil and can wreak havoc on the body. And then there's the fact that crying is a way we demonstrate our humanity to each other: we are the only species that cries in response to sadness or frustration. Plus, crying and showing our emotions helps us to bond with each other.

Huh.

When we release trauma, it gives our systems more energy to get on with everything else. Imagine carrying a really heavy box. Once you've put the heavy box down, it's much easier to think about what you need at the shops, right? If you take the heavy box to the supermarket, all you can think about when you're walking around the aisles is *Christ, this box is heavy*. It's hard to focus on what's the best wine to go with chicken.[4]

After my first attunement, I went to a few local "reiki shares" with the same group. This means that you all go round to someone's house where they've got maybe two massage beds and a couple of sofas, and everyone gets a reiki treatment for free. You then have a chat about reiki and a cup of tea and a biscuit (I'm sure custard creams were present, though my memory has lapsed on this vital detail).

I liked it. My experience of reiki was different every time, too – sometimes I found it relaxing, sometimes emotional, sometimes trippy – and I'd see flashing colours, hear voices, see faces or visions, or go to sleep (I have snored on many massage tables) and have really weird dreams until someone woke me up. The people in the group were relentlessly ordinary, too – mums, mechanics, retired ladies, small business owners. I remember one fleece-wearing woman in her sixties called Margaret giving me a treatment where I felt this huge zap of energy go along my spine. She just giggled and said, "It's better than sex, isn't it, dear!" It was like having a spiritual experience with Miss Marple.[5]

The other thing I realized about reiki after that first attunement was that, as I mentioned earlier, *it's never off*. Sure, you turn it "on" to give a treatment, and you rub your hands together at the end and step away from the client to consciously

---

[4] The answer to this is, in my opinion, anything but that one called "Great with Chicken" – it exists, I've seen it in a supermarket that shall remain nameless. Tesco. Oh, I said it.

[5] Which I am completely in favour of.

"end" the session, but once you have the attunement, those symbols are working within your energy body forever. You will never not have it. And the good thing about *that* is that your system starts to heal itself from the inside, completely independently of your intention. (There are no downsides to reiki – absolutely none.) It will change you, like it or not. And you will always like it.

Over time, these healing energies – and they really are profound – will bring up more and more of your internalized trauma, or energy blockages, or bad vibes you've picked up from a psychic vampire friend – *or whatever* – and heal them. It's a lifetime of clearing, of connecting to the powerful currents of energy through the reiki symbols. Yes, it helps if you use it frequently, but even if you never used it again after your attunement, it would still have a positive effect on your life.

I have also always loved the fact that reiki doesn't give a rat's ass if you believe in it or not; it is completely unmoved by whether anyone believes in energy bodies, God or angels, is a second-degree witch, knows what chakras are, is a Gemini or has a Scorpio rising. No prior belief structure is necessary to receive reiki healing, and no particular beliefs are necessary to give it. It just works. What do I love about reiki? It's easy. It works. There isn't much faffing about.

When I got home from that weekend, I was changed. I felt totally different, as if I'd been altered on a chromosomal level or something equally as pseudoscientific and naff-sounding.

My boyfriend was really annoyed that he'd had to go to a wedding on his own that weekend and he'd had no one to dance with. But I couldn't bring myself to care. I'd just come back from an initiation into a world where, despite some minor things that took me out of my comfort zone, I felt I belonged. I had met people, like me, who were searching for more meaning in their lives, and some other people who had found it and were happy to share their secrets.

I now felt like I was living in a completely different world from him. Interestingly, about a year later, our relationship ended. We had had a nice time together for the most part, but it wasn't right between us. He certainly didn't have the spiritual depth I needed, going forward – not that I suddenly needed to be partnered with a chaos magician to be happy. It wasn't that. But he was someone who was very happy living on the surface, and I was starting to admit to myself that I had always been a deep, hidden-places kind of girl. In fact, I've never had a partner who was into healing or magic (plenty of friends though) – but I have been happiest with the ones who accepted my interest in those things and are/were mature enough to have those deep talks about life, the universe and everything. My journey is my own, but it's nice to be understood – and when you have seen some weird shit and experienced some truly life-altering things, it's jarring and frustrating to be told none of it is real.

In fact, while we're on the subject of relationships, it's not unusual, when you begin the healing path (or any kind of esoteric journey), for things in your life to change; some relationships fall away, sometimes faster than they would usually because you are more aligned with your deeper truths than you were before, and less likely to cling on to things you know aren't working.

Going back to the idea of sound and wavelength, it's also interesting to consider what happens in your life (and certainly in your relationships) when you deliberately change your "vibration" by engaging in healing of some kind. What can happen is that some people drift away, and others are suddenly drawn to you. That's been my experience, anyway. It's as if we all make a sound that's unconsciously detectable to others, and we are all drawn to a similar sound or vibration to our own, or one that is attractive to us because of something we need. We respond, positively or negatively, to the vibrations that others are putting out there.

I had met this boyfriend at a time when my "sound" was something like, "Let's have fun and not connect too deeply about anything!" When I changed my "sound" to "Let's investigate our unconscious fears and talk about death!" he was, understandably, not into it. He was a nice person, I was a nice person (well – I had my moments, anyway), we just didn't mesh anymore.

If you like a good complain, or a good bitch and gossip (and who doesn't, from time to time?), and if you do it a lot, you're likely to attract other bitchy and gossipy people. All well and good, if you're happy. But if you find, after a while, that you feel exhausted by all the drama, change your vibration (change the negative language you use about yourself and others, do some healing, read/watch different TV and books, get off the more toxic social media) and your world will change around you. Same goes for the always down and negative friend who pours cold water on all your good ideas. Now, I'm not saying, "Dump your friend who is suffering with depression!" because that's heartless and not good friend behaviour. But I think we've all known people who aren't depressed but just love being negative for their own masochistic reasons. I would advise waving them on their not-so-merry way, if you can.

As a largely secular society, where many religions don't teach their followers about the needs of the more subtle energy bodies (emotional energy, psychic energy, etc.), we don't understand the need for psychic self-defence. Most people attract and accommodate energy from other people (including negative energies) without knowing that the energy body needs a hygiene practice as much as the physical body does. Imagine if you never bathed or showered. Well, your energetic body also needs cleansing through energetic healing, yogic breathing, etc. When I say "raising your vibration", I mean cleansing first and foremost. Get rid of the little energetic hangers-on a regular basis – by doing reiki, by doing yoga, by meditating, by yogic breathing – and that in itself will make you feel a whole lot better. It will also mean you'll be more able to manifest the good things in your life that you want.

How? Because you're not expending energy on carrying around those energy bacteria you've picked up from other people – or your own trauma – anymore. You can see this in action when people spend too long on Twitter. Stay with me here, this is my very own Gen-X pet theory. Ugh, Twitter. Spending any amount of time on it surely is akin to swimming in thousands of people's weird psychic shit. Then we feel terrible afterwards and wonder why. It's hardly surprising, as a day on Twitter probably attaches several energetic bogeys to your energy system. It makes no difference that it's online: you don't need to stand next to someone to pick up something from them energetically. Thanks for coming to my TED Talk.

When jobs, relationships and situations fall away naturally, let them go. They aren't for you anymore: they're ready for someone else to experience. You have new people to meet, jobs to do and experiences to live. Stagnancy brings unhappiness because the soul – the inner self, whatever it is – knows it is ready for the next thing.

I noticed some friendships falling away when I changed my "vibration" from an exclusively "mom" vibe. I am aware that I do have that natural inclination. I am usually the one who has snacks in her bag and has planned a taxi home. However, I realized that *only* being in this mode – strong, resilient, supportive – wasn't fair to me. Again, this was all part of my unconscious commitment to stoicism and not allowing for my own emotional needs, which made me feel resentful that I was "always solving someone's problems" and "always the sensible one". Violin for one, please! I didn't have to be like that. I chose to be because it made me uncomfortable to be vulnerable. Some examples of how I changed my "vibration": I stopped being a faithful listener to psychic vampires (see above). I also made myself less available to the people who had never put themselves out to see me. I let myself be more outspoken, which is more like my natural personality. Yes, sometimes that meant I inadvertently said "the wrong thing", but I realized that I am a human, and as other people make mistakes and are forgiven, then I should allow myself that margin of error, too. I also weaned myself off the belief that if I didn't buy a lavish gift for someone's birthday then they'd hate me.

Another purposeful thing I did, vibration-wise, some years later, was the terrifying[6] work of allowing myself to be myself, which sounds ridiculous, but is in fact something most of us can struggle with. In my case, in a very small nutshell, I allowed my witchy side to come out and be seen: I posted about my spiritual life on Instagram and I talked about it more in conversation with non-witchy friends, where previously I would have avoided the topic. I think most of us who have made a similar decision will agree that in this situation some people become suddenly less keen on the "new you" (which was always the "you", just hidden before) but others become much more keen. So, it's a kind of "find your tribe" thing, and not a bad thing at all.

For me, one side of "raising your vibration" is the cleansing and protection side, but the other is returning to the self in an authentic way. Sometimes when people talk about "raising your vibration" I feel like their implication is mooning about with some crystals or going to a festival and walking around barefoot eating quinoa. That's all very well, but surely the most radical act of positive, energy-raising change you can perform is to a) truly know the things you want to do, b) do the things you truly want to do, c) be the person you truly want to be and d) most importantly, fuck anyone who tries to stop you (providing all of the above doesn't involve you doing something truly heinous).

Plus, it meant that in those friendships that fell away, I wasn't allowing the other person to be the "mom" – that is a controlling behaviour in itself. Sometimes, we are wise; sometimes, we are stupid assholes. No one is one or the other all the time, and it's nice, though difficult, to be honest about that.[7]

---

[6] I don't mean terrifying as in zombie flesh-eating movies, but more like sometimes the simplest acts of honesty and expressing your truth are terrifying, especially when they lead you to risk losing people you thought were friends.

[7] Except Keanu, who is perfect. Sigh.

I needed – and am now very thankful to have – friendships where I can be a total fuckup and it's okay. I can't say I have that open, okay-to-be-less-than-perfect relationship with many people, because I take a long time to trust others. And, yeah, I *do* love being in control. Who doesn't?

Yet, I have some amazing people in my corner, and I can see that the reason I think they're amazing is that they've fucked up in their lives – often big time – and come back from it. It took me a long time to realize it but, incredibly, this is also the thing that other people love and respect about me.

HA! The irony.

Reiki has been there for me, in the background, for 17 years now, and I genuinely believe it's helped get me through the worst times in my life. Sometimes I wonder where I'd be if I'd never gone to that manky community centre on the Finchley Road for that first free session. But I did, and I guess that day I held up some sort of white flag to the universe, unwittingly surrendering to its gentle and not-so-gentle ministrations on the path to healing.

When I spoke to Gillian Ellis, the reiki teacher who did my Reiki Master training and attunement, she told me much the same thing: that reiki helped her through some of the most difficult times in her life. Gillian is a remarkable woman, and very like many spiritual teachers I've known: friendly, unassuming, living a completely normal life in an anonymous suburb. Yet she has an aura of power, peace and gentleness that comes from years of spiritual practice and dedication.

Interview with Gillian Ellis, Reiki Master

What is reiki?
The word "reiki" is Japanese and it means "divinely guided universal energy". This energy is a vibration that people can tune into through a process from a Reiki Master. Once attuned it is readily available all the time. It works on the physical, spiritual

and emotional levels of self to bring them into balance. We are vibrational beings who draw vibrations to us all the time. We are like magnets.

How does it work?

If you're receiving reiki or have been attuned to reiki, it overrides your personal vibration. If your personal vibration is low, it will bring in a higher vibration. Reiki has been scientifically proven to bring in a vibration higher than pain, which is how it can help with pain. The reiki has a consciousness of its own and finds the areas in the body that need to be balanced – it doesn't need to be consciously directed; it goes where it needs to go.

When you're attuned to reiki, what happens is that the attunement works in the subconscious. It puts a programme in the subconscious so that when someone thinks about reiki, it sends out a signal. I always explain to people that it's like pressing a light switch.

What's it like to receive a reiki treatment?

You can be in a sitting or lying position. During the treatment, you get into a very deep relaxation. You don't need to breathe or think in a certain way when you receive it – all you need to do is lie down or sit down. I've had people come in and say, "I can't relax. I'm not someone who can let go." But it doesn't matter who you are or what you think. The reiki will work on you. People start to relax. They lie down, and I start on the head usually because it helps the mind to relax. You're working on the chakra system: the reiki will help to balance the chakras but the reiki will also help the person to relax the physical body.

Some people will feel a deep relaxation and that's all they get out of it, but I know it's working on different levels at once. Later on, they might have something come to mind that will trigger a realization or help them work through some feelings that they needed to deal with. I've had the experience of people coming to see me with a bad back or trapped nerves, and reiki has un-trapped the nerves and made that pain go away.

After the treatment, I remind them to drink lots of water and flush out all the toxins that the reiki will have released in the body. I also like to support clients after I see them, so I do a follow-up and check in with how people are.

How did you first come to reiki?

I was always interested in alternative therapies and was brought up in a fairly open-minded family, but it wasn't until I had my children that I really began on this pathway. My daughter had eczema as a child and I had to find somebody to help me – doctors were no help. Anyway, I found a herbalist who was able to help. I used to sit in the waiting room while my daughter was having her treatment and talk to her other clients – this woman did a variety of healing techniques including energy work.

I myself was really depleted at the time because I was so exhausted looking after my daughter – I didn't have a good night's sleep until she was three or four because of the eczema. When the herbalist helped her, I was really inspired and I wanted to give back to others in the same way. I wanted something that could help me maintain my own energy levels as well as helping others, and so when I was invited to a seminar about reiki I thought it sounded really interesting, and afterwards, when I had a free taster session, I could really feel the energy coming through when the woman put her hands on my back. So, I signed up from there!

Can you tell me about one particular experience in your personal healing journey that was really meaningful?

When I had my first attunement I felt like I was coming home. I'd always felt I was on the periphery before, and now I found a load of people who had the same kind of interests as me. I was forty at the time and I really felt that I'd found the reason I was put here on Earth: to give and receive this energy. Then when I did reiki two, I realized that I now had a way to help all the causes I was passionate about in the world too: I could send healing to the environmental issues I cared about, to the people suffering who I felt frustrated I couldn't help. I felt less helpless: I could do something about it.

How has reiki changed your life?
I used to suffer with depression, and since doing reiki I've never been depressed. I didn't have that mental battle going on with another world that wanted to take me over. I'd had postnatal depression, though I never asked for help with it. After I had my second child, I could feel it coming back, but when I started with reiki, it went away. I was so relieved: I had two children; I didn't have the time to be depressed!

Then, about two or three months after I was attuned to reiki one, I had the proof that reiki really worked. My mother fell down the stairs and dislocated her shoulder and cut her leg open. She didn't break anything, but she was eighty at the time. My daughter was four and my son was eight and it was the beginning of the school holidays.

I went in the ambulance with Mum and gave her reiki, just to help her keep calm and help her natural healing along. The doctor said that with a dislocation like this, we had one chance to get it back in or they'd have to operate. They asked me if I wanted to come into the operating room with her. I thought, *Well, I'm not particularly squeamish!* So I was in the room while they put her shoulder back in place. You can beam reiki; you don't have to actually have your hands on someone – so that's what I did! No one knew what I was doing. Her shoulder went back in straightaway, which for an eighty-year-old was unusual.

Within six weeks the shoulder had healed, which the doctors were amazed by. She didn't take painkillers at all; I was giving her reiki every day. Her leg healed up nicely and she had no trauma from the accident – often people of that age have emotional trauma, shock, from an event like that, but she was absolutely fine and she was back driving within three months. At eighty some people might never get over an accident like that but she was back to her normal busy life. The other thing was that the reiki managed to keep me calm while I was looking after the kids on the school holidays and looking after Mum. In fact, we had a lovely summer and I really felt like I wouldn't have got through that if I didn't have the reiki. There have been so many other occurrences too, but I can really say that it's changed my life in so many ways, all for the good.

CHAPTER 3

THEY FUCK YOU UP, YOUR MUM AND DAD (AND YOUR GRANDPARENTS, AND YOUR GREAT-GRANDPARENTS)

What is emotional trauma? We've got this far and edged around the idea, but let's think about it for a moment.

From a psychological standpoint, emotional trauma happens when either a person is involved in a current traumatic situation (anything from the death of a loved one to experiencing war, childbirth difficulties, baby loss, a terrorist attack, a humiliating experience, rape, mugging or climate change-related traumatic experiences) or witnesses it (this might include police officers viewing violent crime or abusive video footage, or someone working with the survivors of sex trafficking or some similar support role). It also refers to historic trauma experienced in childhood that an adult may (or may not) have blocked from their memory, but which is causing problems in their adult life. Last, something that causes ongoing stress, such as a heavy workload or a stressful relationship, can cause trauma. Any of these experiences can also lead to PTSD (post-traumatic stress disorder).[1]

The symptoms of trauma can include depression, re-experiencing the traumatic event in flashbacks, insomnia, emotional detachment, loss of self-esteem, despair, self-destructive behaviours (i.e. drug taking and alcoholism), panic attacks, nightmares and intense anger among many others. Conventional treatments for trauma and PTSD currently include cognitive behavioural therapy (CBT)[2], medication and counselling.

The holistic point of view agrees that trauma is caused by difficult life situations, but differs in the way that it conceptualizes what trauma does to a human being. In a variety of therapies, trauma is considered to be psychically "held" in the body and the energy field around the body, rather than just inside the brain, as in the more conventional psychological view.

The energetic model of healing explains that we are made up of a number of linked "bodies", with the physical one being the densest. The physical body is (of course) visible to the eye. Around that, the emotional body surrounds us for several inches, followed by the mental and then psychic body in similar layers, growing ever more subtle in terms of vibration. When people see auras around the bodies of others, they're seeing the denser levels of the energy body, most likely the emotional or mental energy body, often dominated by the colour of the chakra that person is most "in" at that time.

---

[1]   More information about PTSD can be found here: www.nhs.uk/mental-health/conditions/post-traumatic-stress-disorder-ptsd/overview/

[2]   Cognitive behavioural therapy (CBT) is a talking therapy that can help you manage your problems by changing the way you think and behave. CBT is based on the concept that your thoughts, feelings, physical sensations and actions are interconnected, and that negative thoughts and feelings can trap you in a vicious cycle. Unlike some other talking treatments, CBT deals with your current problems, rather than focusing on issues from your past. It looks for practical ways to improve your state of mind on a daily basis. For more information: www.nhs.uk/mental-health/talking-therapies-medicine-treatments/talking-therapies-and-counselling/cognitive-behavioural-therapy-cbt/overview/

When disease or some other bogey (I used bogey earlier, and I'm going to stick with it) comes our way – be that some negative energy or a virus or a traumatic experience – the energetic model states that it will make its way in from the psychic energy body, to the mental, to the emotional and finally the physical, where it will manifest as actual disease or pain. Similarly, when we heal, the bogeys are sent back out through the system in the same way.

I was taught an interesting concept about the healing of the physical body under this rationale, which is that the dis-ease[3] (symbolizing a virus/bacteria/trauma, etc.) makes its way out of the physical body from the core and out to the extremities before continuing to depart through the emotional, mental and psychic bodies. For example, an illness might begin with sickness (core), but as the healing body pushes out the intruder, it becomes a rash that starts at the chest, moves down to the legs and then out through the toes and feet. It's an interesting theory (and I'm not sure if it's got the scientific seal of approval) but I have found it very useful to think about how people's symptoms often morph over time.

Sometimes an emotional problem can even become a physical one or, sometimes, when emotional problems are dealt with, then physical symptoms disappear.

Following the energetic model to its logical conclusion, dis-ease will continue to go deeper into the body until it hits the bones and the internal organs, causing more serious complications. From a holistic viewpoint, then, it makes sense to ward off the nasties before they get that far, with regular deep healing of trauma as well as psychic self-protection.

A reiki practitioner might see, sense or feel trauma as a sticky black substance in someone's aura, or feel fear held in a particular chakra or part of the body. They might even perceive it as a sound or a coldness or sort of manic buzzing feeling – it would be individual to the person giving the treatment.

---

[3] My first Reiki Master, Pennie, introduced me to the use of the word in this way: literally disease as a lack of ease in some way.

However the therapist experiences it (or they might not experience it at all), the idea is that with reiki (or with other related modalities) we are looking to help the client release trapped energy, guiding or propelling the stuck energy back out through the subtle energy bodies.

There is another kind of trauma that therapists are beginning to consider now, which is called inherited, ancestral or generational trauma. What?! Like we don't have enough of our own crap to deal with, we also have to heal our grandparents'? What is life?!

The idea is that the traumas our forebears experience are stored somewhere in our DNA and passed down to us if left unhealed. The science is murky on the details of exactly where the trauma is stored, DNA-wise, but from an energetic healing point of view, it would be stored in the energy body and transmitted through a kind of energetic link between the generations. From my own personal observations, ancestral trauma definitely exists. In my view, it's a combination of energetically transmitted emotion passed through some kind of ancestral link, as well as the cumulative psychological effect that traumatic events have on the family as a unit, which then have an effect on the following generations' behaviour.

For example, children born to parents who experienced rationing during or after World War II might not directly experience rationing themselves, but they still live with a parent who, perhaps traumatized by food scarcity and living in a fear-based attitude toward food, now stockpiles it "in case of emergency". Perhaps then that child takes on some of that trauma-inspired behaviour around food, either stockpiling or having another unhealthy relationship to it. Is this ancestral trauma, or learned familial behaviour? In a way, I don't think it matters how it happens; we can still have these unhealthy patterns we have learned, or have been born with, that we must heal in our own lives.

I have always "felt" my grandmother's traumatic experience as a young woman when she had to leave her home in

Germany in the 1930s to live in England. Her parents – my great-grandparents – feared Hitler's rise to power and, while they stayed behind, my grandmother had to leave the country she loved. Until then, she had lived an idyllic life, roaming wholesomely around the hills and forests and singing with her group of friends as they marvelled at the wonders of nature, just like Maria in *The Sound of Music* (except for the nun bit). Her family lived in a house in a forest and their two pet Alsatians would walk the children through the forest to school every day (to protect the children from tramps, apparently), and then wait for them at the edge of the forest all day to walk them home.

My grandmother was forced to leave her family and her home and friends, and she and her brothers and sisters were scattered to the wind as they emigrated to the UK, Australia and Canada. I remember being shown heavily blacked-out letters from Grandmother to her family back home, covered in the Nazi swastika and warnings in German, as she desperately tried to stay connected to them. Unfortunately, eventually my great-grandfather was taken to a concentration camp, although my great-grandmother was not.

England must have been a kick in the teeth for Grandmother: it was goodbye to a blissful life in the hills and forests, and hello to cramped living conditions, terrible food, dismal weather and a nation that was soon at war with her own. Grandmother had to pretend she was Dutch because many people at the time hated Germans, including her own batshit-crazy mother-in-law who tried to murder her on at least one occasion by baking her a cake with rat poison in it.

Ah, wartime Britain.

Nevertheless, Grandmother stayed, met an English boy, had a family and joined the local Labour Party. She had a difficult marriage with my grandfather who had fought in World War I and never got over it. She died young, almost paralysed with crippling arthritis. Did I inherit some of her trauma? Did my mum and her brothers and sisters? Looking at their lives and mine, I think so.

I had my first BodyTalk treatment around the time my son was two. A friend of mine had recommended it to me – she'd been astounded by the results she'd had after a treatment. I wasn't quite sure what to expect when I rocked up to a local alternative therapy clinic, but my friend had told me all about how the therapist, Maria (also not a nun), had helped with a lot of old family stuff that had been playing on her mind. Plus, she felt great, as if a weight had been lifted from her shoulders. Never one to say no to a new therapy, I booked a session. By that time I'd been using reiki in my life for many years but I knew there was still a lot of deep stuff I needed to heal, somehow, and I had begun to suspect that not all of it was strictly *mine*. It was a few years on from losing my mum to cancer and I felt I had powered through the worst of that grief, but there was still a lot of residual guilt there and a feeling that I hadn't really let her go yet.

Also, I was absolutely shattered from having a two-year-old, and the prospect of lying down for an hour was too much to resist.

Maria – who I still see for BodyTalk sessions about twice a year – is an incredibly calm and zen woman, and, like all my favourite mystics, healers and magicians, is totally grounded in her normal life as well as crazily, beautifully connected to the profound energies of the world. Immediately, I felt at ease when she led me into a cosy treatment room.

She invited me to lie down on a treatment couch. I readily accepted. There was some incense burning, and perhaps a candle. The room had posters of the chakras and energy bodies on the walls. This was all familiar ground from my experiences with reiki.

Maria asked me why I'd come. I didn't have that much of an answer, just that I'd heard good things and I thought I probably needed it. Maybe? Possibly? I think it's an important thing to note here, by the way, that you don't need a watertight, detailed reason to have healing. We all need it all the time: just being human is reason enough. Don't ever persuade yourself out of having any kind of healing because you don't think you have a good enough reason to have it, or you aren't sick enough, or dysfunctional enough. Believe me, we are all deeply in need of it.

Maria explained that my treatment would consist of me talking to her, or her asking questions, and testing my body's responses by feeling a point on my arm for involuntary movements. She would let my body and mind "talk" to her in this way, as well as psychically "viewing" images and messages from me in her imagination to help diagnose any issues. She would then respond to those issues with a variety of techniques including tapping, visualization and even giving me reiki healing if I needed it.

There are similarities between BodyTalk and emotional freedom technique (EFT), which uses tapping movements on certain parts of the body to relieve stress, a little like acupuncture. However, in BodyTalk, the tapping is less to release stress directly and more to "programme" new patterns into the brain, heart or perhaps a chakra that needs to realign to heal itself. Like reiki, the aim of BodyTalk is to straighten out things that have gone wonky so that the body, mind and energy bodies can heal themselves.

The experience itself was nice, but not deeply relaxing in the way that reiki was. Quite often when I received reiki, I'd just nod off (again, two-year-olds will do that to you). However, I was deeply impressed with Maria's depth of knowledge of all the body's physical systems – the endocrine system, nervous systems, brain, meridians, chakras, muscle groups and organs. If anything puts me off training to be a BodyTalk practitioner myself, it's the intensive biology knowledge you have to amass. And that's not even taking into account Maria's understanding of other spiritual systems and practices – from Ayurveda to Buddhism – all of which can be integrated into BodyTalk if the patient needs it.

During my first session, Maria asked me about my mum. I explained that she'd passed away. Maria asked if I'd ever had any ailments on the left side of my body. I said yes, ALL of them. I'd had a bad left knee, sciatica down my left-hand side when I was pregnant, intense headaches on the left side of my head only. Everything that happened to me for a while always happened on my left side.

"Ah," Maria said. "What you have there is the Mother Wound."[4]

I had actually come across this idea before. It's a psychological term for adults who have, as children, not received the nurturing that they need from their mothers, or their mothers have been absent in some way. The Father Wound relates to the same issue with fathers.

"Interestingly," Maria added, "you are also carrying ancestral trauma here, related to your grandmother or even further back. There's something here about being separated from family. There's also a real frustration here you're carrying, an anxiety about being 'the little woman' and not being able to express yourself or have the freedom you should have had. It's actually not yours; you're carrying it from way back. So let's heal that and let it go now."

This chimed in deeply with my knowledge of my grandmother's life – that she had to leave her family and lose the support of her own mother – as well as my mum's life, as she lost her own mother when she was in her early 20s. Both women had had their own children without their mothers being present; this too had now happened to me, having had my son four years after my mum passed away.

The feelings about being the "little woman" and being unfairly repressed also struck a huge chord with me. From my earliest memories I can remember being furious about being regarded as less powerful because of being a woman, which is odd because I don't really know where I might have picked up the idea. I remember telling my dad when I was about six that I was a feminist. Now, bear in mind that this was the early 1980s

---

[4]   There are lots of books and articles you can find on this topic. *Psychology Today* has this useful introduction: www.psychologytoday.com/us/blog/addiction-and-recovery/201910/the-mother-wound and Dr Mari Kovanen's website has this article: www.drmarikovanen.co.uk/healing-mother-wound-healing-emotional-absence/

and feminism was definitely happening, but my mum didn't think of herself as one (she was, though) and certainly didn't talk about feminism to me. So where did I get that rage? Was I responding to some kind of ancestral trauma?

I know from my aunt and my mum that my grandmother felt huge frustration at the fact she kept getting pregnant (my grandfather refused to use contraception or let her use it) and so was a full-time housewife and mother of five (she was also one of five children herself – repeating patterns again). Bearing five children that lived, as well as a number that didn't, must also have been a huge strain on her body, let alone rearing five children. Five! Just imagine it. It makes me bone-tired just thinking about it.

In fact, we would now view my grandfather's behaviour regarding contraception as abusive. My grandmother was bearing children against her will, even though she loved them when they came. I feel instinctively that's the kind of energy that children pick up on and store away in their subconscious. Was Grandmother angry about her continued enforced motherhood? Very probably. Was her life what she had dreamed of as a young woman, roaming the forests and the hills with her friends? It was not. Was her beloved country ruined by an evil dictator? Yes. Had she passed on those negative emotions to us in some way? Quite possibly.

Maria then explained another idea that I've kept as central to my approach to all healing, which is that *healing goes both ways*. The idea is that when you heal, it goes back seven generations and forward seven generations, too; so if you have ended up with some ancestral trauma, then in fact your healing from it ricochets back AND forward like an amazing, high-vibrational tennis game. Kapow! LOVE-LOVE! Forgive the tennis pun.

I've also seen many examples of healing from one side of a rift between two people, radiating to the other person and then from them too, sometimes even out to a group. So when one person decides to engage with healing, it's actually something that affects the whole (and by that I mean, ultimately, the planet and universe and all reality. Woooo!). Like that chaos effect thing about a butterfly flapping its wings in Patagonia which results in you choosing a strawberry yoghurt with your lunch. It's kind of like that, but less cause and effect and more of a "if you heal, the world heals" deal.

Another good reason to get healing.

After my first BodyTalk session I had an incredible dream. I was walking around inside my own brain, only it didn't look like a brain. It was actually quite similar to the Oval Office offices in the TV show *The West Wing*, if you've seen it – a series of interconnected rooms with lots of people walking around briskly, having important, amusing and philosophical conversations and drinking coffee. In one room, a group of actors, including someone in a David Bowie outfit and face paint,[5] gave me a huge cheer and congratulated me on acting out my role in life so far. They were all very impressed by my performance, but also told me that it was time to take off the mask. In the dream, I realized I was wearing one.[6] In another room, Colin Firth reminded me that we had both been very much in love once, but that it was time to move on.[7] And in another room, I joined my mum on an aeroplane on our way to New York where we were going to start a new life.

I took the final part of the dream as a combination of witnessing my mum "passing over" (I do have lots of dreams with people on trains and planes, and it has occurred to me more than once that maybe in my sleep I'm a kind of unpaid helper to the dead), and thereby helping me let her go, and perhaps witnessing my own ability to cross over into the next

---

[5]   Sadly, even in my dream I knew it wasn't actually Bowie. I miss him.

[6]   I think this meant that I had to stop pretending to be a person I wasn't. In my case, I think I was pretending to be someone normal who *wasn't* really into magic, healing and witchy shit.

[7]   I took this to mean that it was time to move on from people in my past that I'd been in love with. However, I'd like to state for the record that I never did have a romantic entanglement with Colin specifically, but I did have a brief crush on him when he was in *Bridget Jones's Diary*.

world too. Whatever, it was an amazing dream. What I loved about it most was literally seeing my brain sorting itself out after the BodyTalk had started realigning it.

Over the years I've had other big dreams as a result of BodyTalk, and I've found that it's helped me hugely in my healing process. In the months after my first treatment, I did feel myself releasing that fear of being "the little woman" in my own relationship, which had frequently come up as a point of tension before. I would accuse my husband (totally unfairly) of treating me in a sexist way and being some kind of terrible patriarchal oppressor, which, in our relationship, is totally laughable. I mean, I control the TV remote at all times[8] and I can count on one hand the times he's ever won an argument. I did very much let that go, and felt happier for it. That had actually never been true in any of my romantic relationships, but it's my belief that my brain may have made me think it was happening because of this inherited fury, this frustration from grandmothers before.

Huh.

Interview with Maria Wilson, BodyTalk practitioner

What is BodyTalk?

BodyTalk is a consciousness-based healthcare system, or an energy medicine. We work on the premise that the body heals itself, and as practitioners, we're trained to observe what is going on within the body-mind of the client. Body-mind means that the body as a whole is intelligent and can talk to us, not just the brain. We tune into the subconscious of the client using a muscle test and a specific protocol of questioning we ask that gives us yes-and-no responses from the muscle we are touching – which is usually on the arm.

---

[8]   This, perhaps more than anything, is surely the ultimate feminist laurel wreath.

So when we use the muscle test we're asking the body, what "section" or system is the imbalance in?

Intertwined with that we have the intuition of the practitioner and any other tools they have as well – other experiences or healing modalities they may have will come into that session. So, BodyTalk in and of itself isn't a closed system. It's totally open and we incorporate so many other influences with it – such as yogic and Ayurvedic philosophies – and then for example I also use reiki as part of it.

So, every session is unique to the person giving it who may come along with their own particular skillset alongside the BodyTalk framework, and unique as well because of the client's own needs and makeup. Everyone has a unique blueprint, if you like – their genetics, their parents, their upbringing, culture, environment, their emotions. Everything, really.

How does it work?

We are also the sum of our belief systems and our programming, which is something that we will often undo for people. So in that way, BodyTalk is almost a negative practice because we undo programming sometimes that has run its course or has stopped being useful. That allows the person to be more centred, grounded, more like themselves. I always use the analogy of a lightbulb covered in paint. If our true self is the lightbulb underneath, we have all these layers of paint on top – all those belief systems and all that programming we've picked up in life. Your body and its innate wisdom – that part of you that knows how to heal you – knows what needs to be balanced and released and in what order, therefore removing those layers of paint and getting back to you being your true self. So, as a consciousness-based healthcare system, what we're doing is really allowing people to remember who they are.

What's phenomenal about the BodyTalk system is that whatever symptom you might bring into the session, and whatever the client thinks they need, the body will tell the practitioner what actually needs to be balanced. Sometimes a client may come in with a painful knee, but we may need to balance a meridian or an emotional release or even something coming from another part of the body. We're guided to do those balances, and as a consequence, the knee repairs itself.

What's it like to have a treatment?

You lie down on a treatment table, fully clothed, and relax. Sometimes I put music on because it adds to the relaxing atmosphere, and music is a frequency in itself, so that can help with the healing.

The way the body works – from the perspective of the head brain, for example – is that the hypothalamus is always scanning the body and keeping the equilibrium within it. When I say head brain, I'm referring to the theory of the body that says we have three sentient "brains": the brain, the gut and the heart. All of those centres have knowledge and regulate what's going on in the body as a whole. By linking into the subconscious, the brain is able to show us what imbalances are in place – which are identified by the hypothalamus. Now, those imbalances can be anything from a physical organ to something in the endocrine system or any other body part; it could be emotional or it could go to an energy system. It might be a belief system, it might be in the circulatory system. So when we're doing the questions and the muscle response, the body is responding by twitching the muscle as we progress down into the specifics of where the issue is.

Sometimes, we go off the books, as it were, and it's not in the body at all – it might be a past life, it might be energetic and outside of the client. But then, on the other hand, if we consider that everything "outside" in terms of the environment is only ever coming through the perception of the client – that's how the world exists for us, solely through perception – then there is nothing "outside".

Then, when we've ascertained the issue and brought it into the conscious mind for the client by describing what it is, we'll do some tapping on the top of the head, over the heart and the gut. They're the three "brains" in the body. The head brain we fix, the heart brain is the remembering and the gut brain is the processing. The tapping "fixes" those formulas for healing into the body, helping it to rebalance itself. Then we go on to the next formula. There's often more than one to do in a session: it depends how much the client can handle, and, as I say, we work very intuitively there and let ourselves be guided by the client. I might give some reiki healing as part of a treatment too.

Permission is a big thing in a treatment session. I always ask permission before we start any session, because it may come up that on one of the levels – mental, emotional, physical, spiritual – there might be a block to the client's healing. It's a sign of respect to get permission beforehand rather than just bowling in and assuming that's the case. You see a lot of people out there working with healing modalities where people might say, can you give healing to my friend or brother or sister, without asking them, and that's a serious abuse. Why? Because this is their life and their journey in this existence and they have to learn from all their "stuff". If you're going in there with healing when it's not right, you're going to put them off their track. Sometimes people do not want healing and that's okay.

How did you learn about BodyTalk?

I came into the therapy world with reflexology and reiki. Someone asked me if I'd heard of BodyTalk Access, which was a small programme within the BodyTalk system. It incorporates a set of techniques that anyone can learn. I went along and did this day's workshop, and the techniques were amazing; I practised on myself and on my family and I could really see significant changes on stress levels and general health. I wanted to know more so I booked a session with Karen Best who is one of the English tutors of the BodyTalk system, and I was profoundly blown away! It really felt like I'd come home; it felt so right, and I just thought, *I've got to do this, I've got to train in this.* And I haven't looked back!

So can you tell me one particular experience in your personal healing journey that was really meaningful in some way?

Health-wise, I've experienced migraines, and they're the type of migraines that knock you out for twenty-four hours. They were really bad at one time and they've gone now. But the thing that stands out for me was experiencing a moment of pure bliss.

Everything I've learned in BodyTalk – lots of different trainings – all leads toward personal growth. So I'd come home from various training sessions and tell my husband about what I'd learned. At the time he was obsessed with proving that the things I'd learnt weren't true! He couldn't believe what I was telling him. Yet, ironically, in his own journey seeking the truth, he had an amazing experience of enlightenment, and that was something that I wanted. I was like, how did he get it?! It wasn't fair. I was the one doing all the training.

One day, I was out walking the dogs and I'd climbed this hill. I was standing at the top and I was basking in the sunlight – there was a lovely breeze and all that – and something happened, and I was suddenly in a moment of bliss. In that moment, it was like my heart centre had totally opened up and I'd let go of everything. I was physically on the ground but I felt like I was lifted. It was a magical moment. I think it's something that can happen when you're grounded and centred but have also let go of so many belief systems. You realize you have a higher self: there's more to us than the human body, and that connection is where this bliss state can come in.

It only lasted five minutes and then my phone rang. Ha! But that was enough.

How has BodyTalk changed your life?

BodyTalk was the first thing that really introduced me to the idea of consciousness. That we are more than our body. Even with the training I'd done before, I never really understood that. And then with maybe ten years of BodyTalk training, including all those moments of personal development, I was able to bring those experiences to my time with clients and help them to see there's more than just what we see. It's almost like it's taken me from a 3D world to a 5D world.

CHAPTER 4

CRYING WHILE THE SPIRITS WATCH: BEREAVEMENT AND MY EXPERIENCE OF SPIRITUAL HEALING

I'm aware that I've promised you some hilarious tales of bawling my eyes out in random locations and, so far, they haven't appeared that much yet. Those strange places ARE coming, I promise. Bear with me.[1]

Like many people, I lost my mother to cancer. She had fought it bravely, but in the end, after beating breast cancer when she was 50, we discovered that she had bone cancer 10 years later, which spread to most of her organs. She died within about 18 months of her diagnosis.

---

[1] Just to keep you going on the "ridiculous locations" front, please enjoy the story a friend told me about his intense magical order who held rituals above a vegan café in Vauxhall (a not particularly posh area in south London) and kept getting interrupted in their dramatic invocations to the gods by café customers popping to the loo. The story ended up in the *Daily Mail*. As my friend very rightly pointed out, one feels that a more private ritual space might have been optimal.

As you can imagine, this was a terrifically sad time. One of my saddest memories is our last Christmas together: we'd always spent Christmas just the two of us, sometimes with a boyfriend of mine along for the ride, but the best ones were when it was just her and me. We'd get up late, open our presents, eat a box of chocolates before lunch and then make a huge roast turkey lunch just for the two of us. Then we'd watch a classic 80s movie in the afternoon like *Romancing the Stone* (my favourite) or *Indiana Jones and the Last Crusade* (hers).

That last Christmas, I had very little money because I was in the middle of a serious debt crisis, and I'd had to spend the last of my money on the council tax my flatmate of the time had apparently forgotten to pay for a few months. So, I had very little to give Mum in terms of presents. I'd wanted to get her something special because she'd been having such a hard time of it, what with the chemotherapy and the pain, mostly in her spine at that time. (The pain bone cancer causes is horrible; even morphine didn't really relieve it, and her mobility was seriously impaired for those last couple of years.)

So, I couldn't give Mum much and that made me feel awful. Worse, she'd been going to a day hospice for a while, once or twice a week, and at the hospice she'd made me a memory book containing pictures of herself. To remember her by.

As if I could ever forget her face.

It was such a lovely gesture, but it still makes me sad now to think about that book. It makes me sad to think about how you can stand to make something like that for your child, because you know you're going to die. How must it feel to know that, to see death coming so inevitably? Mum always had a kind of toughness to her – she'd learned to be self-sufficient, even though she was such a kind and sweet person – but even for those who have learned to be tough, facing death is almost impossible. I remember one day quite soon after we'd been told she had bone cancer – and what the life expectancy was – I was sitting at the dinner table with her, watching her try to eat and failing. She was so upset, in such a state of panicked desperation, she just couldn't get her throat to work at all. She just didn't know what to do with herself.

Even as an adult, it's terrifying when you see a parent at their lowest ebb; when they can't parent anymore, and when they're struggling to get through the day as a vaguely together human being. I felt angry again at that point, when the cancer came back: I was angry at the cancer, and I was angry at Mum because the child in me was shouting BUT YOU'RE THE ONE WHO'S SUPPOSED TO MAKE EVERYTHING OKAY. JUST MAKE IT OKAY. MAKE IT OKAY FOR ME.

I was angry. I was so, so angry. And I had to realize that sometimes, you can't make things okay. Sometimes, terrible things happen and no one can or will protect you from them. That's just the truth about life: it can be beautiful, and easy, or low-key difficult, and relentlessly hard, and sometimes there come times that are so inevitable and brutal you barely believe they'd be allowed to happen. And yet, they do.

It was a very difficult year. When Mum was in hospital, I was shuttling back and forth from London to see her as much as I could while holding down my job, my flat and my spiralling debt problem. When I would see her, I'd give her as much reiki as I could, spending nights and days at her bedside as her condition deteriorated. Once, I remember sitting in the room she was in with one other woman and them both falling asleep once I started the reiki. That was when we could still have conversations and a laugh now and again.

In the last weeks, she lost her speech and her sight, and because the cancer was now in her brain, she was living in what must have been a terrible delusional state. She was terrified of things we had no way of understanding, often crying out in pain and distress. It was a gruelling, savage thing to witness, and I wouldn't wish a death like it on anyone. I remember one day leaving the hospital, going back to the car park and weeping in the car. At that point I just wished that the end would come. There was no quiet slipping away for her, no gentle slope into dreaming. There was only pain and horror, and I was exhausted.

I remember calling my friend and bawling down the phone, and her asking gently, "Where are you? Come over; don't go home on your own. Can you drive, or shall I come and get you?"

I have always been blessed with amazing, caring friends, and they held me up every time I couldn't stand on my own.

When Mum passed away, it was a mixture of relief at not having to sit in the hospital anymore, grief and shock, and a weird kind of blankness. I organized the funeral, wrote and delivered the eulogy, tied up all her official paperwork, closed her bank account, stopped her incapacity benefits and did the thousand and one other jobs you have to do when someone dies.

After I'd done all that, the grief really rolled out. It was like being steamrollered. I couldn't leave the house. I left my job as I just couldn't cope with working; getting out of bed was a problem, never mind having to talk to people, do the commute, concentrate. I hardly slept, and cried almost constantly.

Rather than do nothing, I enrolled myself on an MA which only required me to attend a class for four hours a week – that, I could just about cope with, and I wanted something that would keep my mind busy. Amazingly, in this time, I also managed to maintain a relationship with my boyfriend (who would become my husband) who I'd met before Mum died. He saw me through it all and never once wavered, supplying hugs and cups of tea and listening to me in the middle of the night. In retrospect, I'm not sure what he got out of it. But he saved my life.

As it was, my mind strayed to some very dark areas in that first year after Mum's death. I became fixated on death. I couldn't get thoughts of decaying flesh out of my mind. I thought obsessively about rotting meats. I became convinced that my flat's bathroom was haunted. I felt split into many parts, as if my spirit had been totally shattered. Being around other people made me feel paranoid, attacked, possessed by evil spirits. I also became convinced that I too was going to die soon and was preoccupied with thoughts of suicide, in a if-it's-going-to-happen-anyway-might-as-well-hurry-it-along kind of way. There were times during the two years after Mum's death that

I could only find a sense of peace by planning my own death. Obviously, I didn't do it. But there is a kind of place you can get to, I found, where even something as dark as that provides you with a sense of control that you don't feel you have elsewhere, and with relief that soon all the pain will be over.

I was, at the time, actually terrified that I was going mad. I was so convinced that if I went to the doctor and told them what I was experiencing, they would lock me up in a mental hospital and throw away the key.

Now that I'm sane and healthy (ha! More or less) I know that it's highly unlikely anyone would have sectioned me at the time, and probably the doctor would have referred me to a bereavement counsellor and possibly prescribed some short-term antidepressants. But, at the time, my judgement severely impaired, I decided that I did need some help but that it would be on my terms, so I found a spiritual healing therapist specializing in bereavement, and off I went to see her instead.

Now, very unfortunately, I have lost this lady's name, and so I can't recommend you to her here. I do remember that she lived in Forest Hill in south London at the time, and that I went to her house for a few sessions during which I basically cried my heart out.

This woman, let's call her Sheila (her name definitely wasn't Sheila. Claire? Sarah? It's gone), asked me to lie down on her treatment couch and talk to her about why I'd come. I explained that I'd recently lost Mum.

Sheila wasn't using reiki, that I do remember, but she nonetheless channelled what felt like quite similar healing energy around me, and then called in my mum's spirit so that we could experience the closure that I didn't feel I'd had. She asked me to verbalize what I wanted to say to Mum, and I did my best.

In between vociferous crying (Sheila seemed to take it in her stride) I spoke directly to Mum's spirit, which Sheila told me had appeared: I told her I was sad to lose her but that I understood it was her time to go. I told her I just wished that we'd had more time to have fun together, in my childhood and as adults. When I looked back on our time together, I felt sad that there hadn't been many laughs. There had been plenty of wisdom and talks and spiritual growth – and enough food and drink and a roof over our head – but this is what I'd missed, I told her. However, I was grateful to have had her as a mother. I really was, and I always will be.

Sheila conveyed messages from Mum to me: that she loved me, that she understood, and that she was resting now, but that she would be reincarnating again soon. (I'm stating here and now that, personally, I'll be DONE with Earth when I'm gone and WILL NOT be reincarnating again if I have any choice in the matter. I'll do something else. Run the snack bar on the astral planes or something. All power to my mum who was brave enough to come back for another go.)

It was an emotionally intense experience, but my attitude toward these things has always been that I've paid for the session, or committed my time to being there, so I might as well make the most of it. If you visit a spiritual healer who claims to be speaking to your dead mother, then join in the conversation. What have you got to lose?

In follow-up sessions, we didn't repeat that experience but Sheila worked with me on my obsession with death and decay.[2] I told her about a recurring dream I'd had of being trapped in a murky pond which was full of terrifying, large, shadowy fish. She gave me more healing sessions – similar to reiki, in a fully clothed, hands-on kind of way – and the dreams changed somewhat, with the water in the pond growing clearer and more pleasant.

In the last session we had, Sheila asked me how the water was looking. I remember that at that point the pond had progressed into a number of pools in a nondescript countryside landscape. I was still in one that was a bit murky, but I could

---

[2] Which is, by the way, quite a common experience for people who are bereaved, as is the belief that you will soon die or an obsession with death in general. So if you've experienced this, try not to worry. It will pass. Unless you're in a Death Metal band, in which case it's your professional bread and butter.

see others nearby that were clear and sparkling. That seemed a good omen: if at least I could see better times ahead, then that was a good thing.

Soon after that, my MA course drew to an end and I got a new job. My grief was still intense, but I was over the hump of the worst of it. Slowly, I began to rejoin the living world and leave behind my stay in the world of death.

Interview with Tiffany Wardle, spiritual healer and psychic medium

Hi Tiffany! Can you tell me about what you do?

So, people often come to me for psychic readings but I'm concentrating much more on healing now.

Let's talk about last week. A lady came to me because she'd just lost her son. People come to me and ask me about their dead relatives, and I say, I'm not a medium, I'm here to put your soul back on track. But in the process of putting her soul back on track, we did a healing and we communicated with her son on the other side. And her son did come through and talked about her future. Then we did the healing afterwards.

Nowadays, I do an intuitive healing. I know reiki – I'm a Reiki Master, I trained in Japan. I climbed the mountain where Dr Usui discovered reiki. I learned Lemurian, crystal, even dolphin reiki! Now I just kind of put it all together. Guides come through and sometimes they're doctors or healers that have passed over, and they tell me what's wrong and what to do. My healing has moved on over the years, so I don't have to stick to a routine anymore.

What's Lemurian healing?

I discovered Lemurian healing after I discovered reiki, and I found the two types of healing quite similar, because in both you use different symbols. In Lemurian healing you also have to have the symbols integrated and downloaded into your system by a teacher, the same as reiki. I found I really connected with it because I really connected with Lemuria. I've written books about Lemuria. I was already an energy healer and a psychic, so it made sense to me. I realized also that whatever you call it, all this energy is basically the same – it's all one energy, it's all chi, we're just using it in different ways.

In Lemurian healing there's a symbol for confidence, there's a symbol for protection, joy, one to put you on the path to your soul purpose, and there's an overall master symbol – again, like reiki – which you can use if someone's not asking for anything specific. You have the symbols within you and then you use them on the client, sharing that energy with them.

The client doesn't have to be in front of you. Energy doesn't know if you're next to me or on the other side of the world. So, especially because of Covid, pretty much all of my healing is distance healing.

What's it like for someone to experience a healing from you?

When we do a reading or a healing, I find you get the healing anyway, even when I just do a psychic reading. Within three days of the healing, people tend to feel centred and peaceful, and then get what I call little miracles. They'll get little ideas about what to do next or where to go. Or, random things will happen to them which will mean their career is now on track, or their life partner is going to appear. These doors start to open because the healing goes into the soul, and the soul starts to know which way to go.

The immediate response is a rush of energy. Some people cry as a release, and if that happens then I explain to them what's going on. They may also feel ecstatic, or they may feel a rush of euphoria. So, people respond in different ways. Sometimes it can have very quick results. One day, my dad had a toothache. He'd had it all day. I just put my hand on his jaw and it disappeared immediately. But most people come to me for a deeper reason.

Do you see clients several times, or is once enough?
I never tell people to come back, because what I'm ultimately trying to do is put people's souls back on track. So, hopefully, once is enough – you know you've done your job properly when people don't pick up the phone again – or at least until the next chapter of their life happens. But, saying that, I have to say most people do come back because they move on to the next thing to heal. Like, for the first time it might be love trauma. Then it might be a career or a money block. And healing-wise, once they're attuned to the energy, it's more like a top-up. Like a balloon that deflates a bit and needs a top-up.

Plus, life happens – plenty of trauma-inducing stuff there!
Exactly. That's what I say! If life was perfect, you wouldn't need me.

How did you come to healing in the first place?
I was working for a newspaper. I studied law and then worked in the media for ten years. I was a real business person! I owned properties and my own little business and I thought that was going to be my lane.

I was sitting at work one day and my hands started burning. When I say burning, I mean it was like they were on fire. The pain was excruciating. This carried on until I went to hospital; I'd been to doctors and no one could figure out what was wrong with me. They thought I was allergic to something.

I remember lying awake at night with them burning. I'd put my hands in the freezer or under the cold tap.

It was my mum that said to me, "I think you're a healer." I thought, *What does that mean?* I knew I was psychic from when I was like two or three years old, but that had been completely pushed aside because of academia. So I thought that was all forgotten about. No, it wasn't! The moment I started to learn about healing, the pain went away. It became very obvious that there was an energy that was trying to rush through me, and it was getting stuck in my hands because I wasn't doing what I was meant to do.

The first thing I learnt was reiki, which seems to be the first port of call for many people. The pain went away, and I had the most astonishing experience – which has never happened before or since. It was like I had a total photographic memory. I read the course materials once and I knew it backwards. That's never happened to me! I don't have a photographic memory. In fact, I have a terrible memory! But when it came to reiki, it was like it was all already there inside me.

How did healing change your life?

So then, when I'd just learnt reiki, I bought these spas. And I thought I'll do the healing in the spas, and I'll get some beauty practitioners in to do the rest. I was still in that mode of not believing this new life of healing could earn enough money. I still had that business mindset.

My word, spirit had other plans for me!

I put everything I had into buying these spas. I sold some houses. It took two years. And then the franchise went into administration, and all my money was gone. In one day. In one email! Everything I had.

I had £600 left in the bank. I had no job because I'd been working on this spa plan. I had nothing. And with that £600 I bought a flight to Japan. So I went and sat at the top of the mountain where Dr Usui had discovered reiki. I sat and sat there, and after a while I started to see my grandmother in spirit. I started to get messages, and the message was: *You walk, we'll direct you in life, every step of the way.* I was walking down the mountain as I got that message and I was still so angry about everything I'd lost. But by the time I got to the bottom I was a completely different person.

From that day on – I was 28 then – that's how I've lived. Every step I've taken, I have been shown where to go. But I did absolutely need to lose everything, to strip everything back for it to happen.

I remember being in my flat in Croydon and a message came through: *You will book a flight to Hawaii on 27 April. You're not coming back.* I was like, what? (Laughs) I don't have any money for a flight. What am I going to do when I'm there? But the guides were just like, *you're doing it!*

So I went, because I always do what I'm told now (laughs) and you just have to trust. I spent two years travelling – I'd do three months in LA, two months in Hawaii, California, Arizona, Colorado. I climbed Mount Shasta twice and that's when I got the download to write the second Lemuria book about healing. A guide would show up, and they wouldn't leave me alone until I wrote down what they said.

The first time they showed up, I had no idea it was about me writing a book. I just wrote down whatever they said. I had no idea how to write a book! Then when I'd written down what one of them said, they'd disappear and another one would turn up. That book was published in 2011 and people still ask for Lemurian attunements and healing now.

It's been quite a ride!

CHAPTER 5

HEALING THE WITCH WOUND

When it comes to my favourite locations for transformative healing experiences, my top two are:

1 In a room on an industrial estate above a mechanic's workshop (with the mechanic at work downstairs).
2 On an army base.

This is the army base story: Dawn was recommended to me by a friend who knew her through the witchcraft scene. At the time, I was looking for someone who was a past life regression therapist because I was writing a poetry book about past life memory. I'd always been fascinated by the idea of past lives, and at a very young age – perhaps 12 or 13 – I'd read a book by Edgar Cayce which seemed to make total sense to me.[1] Cayce's channelled

---

[1] Edgar Cayce was an American clairvoyant who claimed to channel from his higher self. Cayce's sessions occurred during a trance state when he would fall asleep. His friend Al Layne, his wife, and later his secretary Gladys Davis Turner, would record his words. During these sessions, Cayce would answer questions on healing, reincarnation, dreams, the afterlife, past-life, nutrition, Atlantis and future events. As a devout Christian and Sunday school teacher, his prophesizing claims were a source of trouble for him because channelling was criticized by practitioners of his faith as being demonic. Cayce believed that it was his subconscious mind exploring the dream realm, where he believed minds were timelessly connected.

messages about reincarnation and the afterlife formed a large part of the beliefs of what would become "new age" spirituality.

Past life regression is based on the belief that we as humans have had lives before this incarnation, and that we will likely reincarnate again after this one. (I personally believe this, though I don't necessarily think it's in a linear timeline. Our current scientific rules of time and space surely don't have to apply after death – so why couldn't we have other lives in other timelines, out of order, as it were? I'm also not discounting experiences in realms other than Earth – why do we always have to be humans? I'm fully open to being a sentient gas in another universe.) The theory behind reincarnation is that each incarnation teaches us something new or brings us closer to perfection/closer to god/makes us a more evolved spiritual being. This was something I was taught from childhood. My mum was a deeply spiritual woman who had a very particular view of life, including reincarnation.

The idea of past life regression or recall is that we can go through a kind of meditative or hypnotic process and tap into a part of our awareness that remembers those other experiences which we would not usually be cognisant of. It's not necessary for us to remember our past lives, and many experts on the subject would say that, in fact, we have a purposeful "forgetting" when we incarnate into a new life so that we can focus on the lessons and experiences in this life rather than be obsessed by the past.

Dawn and I had spoken on the phone and I explained that I wanted to be regressed, as a kind of research for the book, and she'd very kindly agreed to help me out.

One autumnal evening in 2013, I drove over to what was in fact a Territorial Army centre I hadn't even known was near-ish to where I lived (are army bases always in a kind of awareness dead zone? They seem to lurk quietly at the edge of towns and cities, invisible to everyone apart from those that are in the know). I parked up in a designated area and called Dawn on her mobile so she could come and get me.

Amid the concrete and the blocky houses emerged a friendly-looking woman in a fleece and long skirt with a few sparkly scarves draped around her neck. She introduced herself as Dawn and welcomed me into her house on the complex. She lived there with her husband who was involved with the TA. She herself was a witch who had recently been undergoing treatment for a brain tumour. "You've got to forgive me if I forget things, or get muddled," she laughed.

Dawn was also a reiki practitioner, and it was fascinating to consider that here was a woman who was undergoing chemotherapy for a brain tumour, yet who was vibrant, energetic and full of beans. She was using reiki on herself every day, she told me, and the doctors were amazed that none of her hair had fallen out with the chemo, and she'd had minimal pain or fatigue.

I liked Dawn straight away: she was chatty, hilarious and totally down to earth. We had a cup of tea, sitting in her crystal-laden treatment room away from the rest of the small house, and she explained what past life regression was, and how it worked.

First, she took me through a deep relaxation process similar to things I'd done in yoga: I lay down on a massage treatment bed and started deep breathing into different parts of my body, tensing that part fully and then letting it go. Head, neck, chest, arms, core, legs, feet, hands. Then she started leading me in a guided visualization to take me into a deeper, more hypnotic state (although I was aware of my surroundings at all times).

First, she had me imagine I was sitting comfortably on a chair in a beautiful, calming location of my choice. I still remember clearly that I imagined sitting on a deckchair on a grassy cliff, looking out to sea. I relaxed more and more deeply, listening to Dawn. Next, she asked me to imagine I was walking down a long set of stairs. Down and down and down I walked, imagining steps cut into the cliff, like the stairs I remembered from a clifftop castle in Cornwall.

I got into a deeper and deeper meditative state, but I still knew I could "wake up" whenever I wanted to. Next, Dawn told me that I would now come upon a long pathway leading through nature, with a series of doors alongside the path. I imagined walking down the path, looking at the doors, and Dawn told me that I should see the numbers of years on them as I passed.

I was so deep into this meditative state that I saw this pathway and the doors very clearly indeed. The pathway was a neat grey gravelled path that led through an open part of a green forest, and the doors sat on my left as I walked past. I remember how deeply immersed I was in that vision. I really did feel as if I were there, while knowing that my body was back in a little room filled with crystals and Dawn and half-drunk cups of tea on a Territorial Army base in Surrey.

Next, Dawn's voice said, *you'll find a door that you want to open. When you find it, walk through the door and tell me what you see.*

I found a door and walked through it.

I don't remember the year on the door, but as I walked through it, I had a sudden vision of being in a chapel. Dawn's voice said, *If you can't yet see where you are, look at your feet first. What's on your feet? Start from there.*

I looked at my feet, but in fact I didn't have to, because I could see that I was wearing brown leather sandals and also a grey or light blue nun's habit. I was with the rest of my fellow nuns in this chapel, and we were all singing. And it was *beautiful*.

I still remember the heart-bursting joyfulness that I felt, in that vision – was it a vision? A memory? I still don't know – the feeling of being part of this sisterly group, the pure joy of being together. It was a sudden, all-encompassing emotion that came out of nowhere, and which took me by complete surprise. I'd been prepared for the fact that I might see some unusual or interesting scenes, but I hadn't been prepared for the fact that I might have such a deep emotional connection to the things I'd experience.

It was as if, in this life, for some reason I'd forgotten my best friend or the love of my life, and then suddenly they'd walked into the room and I'd remembered them, and felt all the love I had for them sweeping back to me.

That was all there was for that door, but I could feel the tears slipping down my face as Dawn called me back. I didn't want to leave. I was a part of that group and I had this overwhelming sense of purity and togetherness that I had never felt before.

Yet, interestingly, as I left the room, opening the same door I'd come in by, and returned to the walkway, my emotions ebbed away very quickly. I still felt touched by the experience, but I no longer felt desperately sad to have left.

I walked along the walkway, watching the doors disappear off into the distance, until I felt called to open another one.

This time, it felt oddly contemporary. I saw myself as a rather large woman, resplendently dressed in a highly patterned, colourful muumuu, in a suburban house somewhere, though not necessarily Britain. Just from a fashion point of view this felt more like the 60s or 70s. I knew that I was married to an Indian man with a small frame who was very kind and loving and made me laugh a lot. I knew that I loved clothes, did not care a hoot about being a large lady and, quite the reverse, very much enjoyed having a big personality to match. I also suddenly "knew" that in that "life" my adorable tiny husband had died before me, and again the tears rushed back. I really felt the grief of losing this man who I had absolutely adored, and who had adored me. I know it sounds INSANE, but I really felt it. It was heartbreaking. Their love was so pure, and it was honestly like being kicked in the chest to know that I, or this woman, had lost someone so very special.

Dawn gently let me cry and then suggested I find my way out of the door when I was ready. Again, I found that the emotion dissipated on closing the door behind me.

Last, I tried another door, which led me somewhere very different.

I was sitting at the edge of a swamp on a kind of wooden jetty at night or perhaps late dusk. I was alone, and aware that I was usually alone. I knew that I lived nearby, and that I was a bit of an outsider. In fact, I knew that many people didn't like me very much.

That was all there was, but I had a deep sense of magic, of being connected to the natural world, of the swamp, and that this was a kind of in-between place. There was a sense of stillness and acceptance that was very profound. I don't remember the year for this one, but it didn't feel at all recent. It seemed very ancient.

There was a different feeling attached to this one, though, a kind of sadness that was unlike before. It wasn't heartbreak, but more an aloneness.

Dawn started to bring me back then. She had me retrace my steps slowly – along the pathway, up the long stairs, back to my deckchair looking out to sea. I stayed there for a minute or two, resurfacing, and Dawn finally guided me back to opening my eyes, wiggling my fingers and being back in the present.

Afterwards, we talked about what I saw and what Dawn had experienced herself. She told me that in one experience she'd gone back to a time that was like the Stone Age and had seen herself as a naked hairy man who had a bad leg, which we had a good laugh about. All hers were pretty far back in time, she'd said, but there was no reason for it that she could tell, and when I frowned about one of my "visions" looking like it was the 60s or 70s – when I'd been born in the late 70s – she just shrugged and said (a little like I believe now), "We don't really understand quite how it works, but that isn't unusual. Maybe alternate realities? Multiverses? A message from your deep brain? You saw what you saw, so make of it what you will."

One thing we talked about afterwards was what is called by some "the witch wound". Dawn herself had had a vision of being a kind of witch in the past, like a village herbalist, and we talked about my vision on the swamp. I don't know if my vision had been about being a witch myself per se, but it prompted a conversation about women at the margins of culture, in touch with nature, whom we might now term a witch or wise woman.

The concept of the witch wound is that we all hold an ancestral or historical connection to the persecution of witches, which has led in part to a psychological sense of shame about being in our power today. Now, in my opinion, this wound is not limited to those persecuted for witchcraft in the past, but is also connected with those being persecuted for witchcraft today in parts of the world where it is still illegal. And also more broadly to other far-reaching, terrible experiences of persecution by death and torture that humanity has wreaked on itself for reasons of gaining power over particular groups. You might include the Holocaust; the Rwandan genocide; the "ethnic cleansing" (a horrible term) in Srebrenica, Bosnia in 1992–1995; the Cambodian genocide committed by the Khmer Rouge between 1975 and 1979; the partition of India in 1947 when between one and two million people died; and so many more horrific, appalling and nightmarish incidences of the suffering and death of large numbers at the hands of ideologically driven governments obsessed with taking power and identifying certain groups to sacrifice as a means to an end.

Although there are some important differences between the witch trials and the other genocides I've listed, they all point to deep ancestral wounds that (I believe) humanity carries in its soul – a communal soul, if you will, that mourns for our losses and carries the horror witnessed. This ancestral wounding makes us afraid to stand up for what we believe in; it makes us fear our own power. Because look what happens to those who stand up to authority; look what happens when we fight autocratic power. Don't get me wrong – I don't blame any of us for this. What rational person wants to put their head above the parapet? We carry the fear, even if we didn't experience something directly, of someone identifying us as somehow "wrong". Of not fitting in. Of being persecuted by others.

You can watch the news every day and see autocratic power in action: when we see climate protestors murdered in some parts of the world for their activism, their power; when people receive death threats on social media and are afraid for their own lives for speaking their truth in the #blacklivesmatter movement or sharing their experiences with #metoo; when governments persecute certain groups in their countries. It happens everywhere, every day, in some way.

Many times, our instinct is to be angry at those who insist on speaking their truth and being powerful – those refusing to live in a state of fear – because their action challenges our fear, and, man, that is uncomfortable! We do not like being uncomfortable! It sucks! I mean, all we really want is a quiet life, right? I know I do.

The feeling I get is anger (God, it sounds like I'm always so angry! I'm pretty chill most of the time, honestly), a knee-jerk response toward someone or something that my deep self feels is being too much. *Pushing too hard. Not being fearful enough.* To me it's a feeling that says, *Hey, you knew the rules, you chose to break the rules, so don't cry about it now.*

It is a horrible feeling to have. It is deeply non-compassionate toward others and, worse, it assumes that the "rules" are always correct. Always, when I examine the feeling, I realize that my anger is misplaced. I actually really admire that person for their lack of fear, and it's actually about my own fear. It's always about you, folks. You are the centre of your universe.

Heads up: the rules are not always correct. In the case of the Holocaust, what person would rationally say, *Hey, you know what, you knew Hitler hated Jews, so you should have left Germany when you could. Don't cry about it now.*

Right. No one would say that, because not only would it ignore many of the facts about Hitler's rise to power, the limited ability of millions of people of leaving the country with nowhere to go and with international governments' caps on immigration, the knowledge of the concentration camps not even being in the public awareness until 1942 (when emigration for Jews from Germany had been closed), but it would also be a horrendously cruel and insensitive thing to say. No one expects to be murdered for their political views, their religion or the fact that they may or may not have supplied a herbal potion to their neighbour.

You should be able to object to climate change without being murdered. You should be able to live peacefully in your own damn country without being murdered. It's completely okay not to expect or foresee that.

But this is the human psyche, remember. There's all kinds of deep, dark crap in there, and one of those things is fear, a necessary emotion that protects us (argh, a snake!) but that sometimes – often – keeps us from connecting to our full power. I believe that "the witch wound" is a deep-seated, communal fear of persecution, based on the many, many events when it was a reality for millions of humans. That persecution – slavery, apartheid, colonialism – is not made up. It was real, and we feel it.

I think here, since I am delving into world history, persecution and All The Big Themes with a kind of wild and probably inadvisable abandon, I should say that I am by no means trying to appropriate the suffering of other cultures for myself as a white woman living in the UK in 2021. I am horrified by what humans have done to each other over the years, but I would not pretend that the Rwandan genocide, for instance, has affected me or my family directly, and neither have any other of those events (except for the Holocaust, which my grandmother had to leave Germany to escape). My point here is that I believe events like the witch trials and the Holocaust, sit in our collective unconscious like a wound and it is up to us all collectively to heal it, whether that be in an individual, spiritual or practical sense (educating each other, making reparations, listening to the voices and experiences of those who have suffered, trying to create a better world). Or, indeed, by consciously working to avoid the practice of persecution wherever it may exist for us in our lives and replace it with a love for our fellow humans. If you have been privileged enough not to have been personally negatively affected by something, you might want to examine what your role is within the situation. And if you have a more powerful role, or privilege, for example as a white person in a fundamentally racist Western society, or a heteronormative person within a largely heteronormative society, or a neurotypical person within a society that frequently misunderstands and under-represents its neurodivergent members, get on that. This too is a real part of healing "the witch wound", as it were, because we reclaim our power when we stand up for what we believe in.

I personally don't agree that one's spiritual life is separate from one's political life and opinion. I can see why people *do* have that point of view: if you're a Buddhist or a Christian or a pagan and you do your weekly worship, what does that have to do with taxes? What does that have to do with your views on crime or education or climate change? It seems to be separate, right? I guess it depends on your point of view. To me, everything is everything. I take a holistic view, because if your God is all-powerful, and you have a holistic view of being part of everything, and everything is a part of you, if you have a sense of connectedness to nature and all-that-is, then your daily life is your spiritual life and vice versa. You are a spiritual being having a human experience, and that human experience of the world is sacred. Therefore, what you do in your "mundane" life is as much a spell as any actual spellcasting you might do; everything is a prayer, everything is a dedication. I accept that the world, and humans, are not perfect. But I believe in healing as a necessary counterpoint to suffering.

Having power is not a bad thing. I want to say that loud and clear from my vantage point as someone engaged in healing. Now, you might be thinking, *Why the flip are we suddenly talking about power and politics when a minute ago we were past-life-regressing with adorable Dawn at the Territorial Army as her military man husband snoozed in front of the TV next door?*

Well, it's relevant, is why. Because I've wittered on about some of the despicable human atrocities from our collective past, you might be thinking, *Ah, yes, power is all well and good, but surely those millions of deaths are what happens when power is abused. So, is reclaiming our power something we should really be aiming for in our personal healing? You can have too much power, you know.*

Yes. Terrible things have happened in the world because of the abuse of power. But there are different kinds of power.

I always look at our popular media – TV and films – which often has the theme of "power corrupts" somewhere: evil god Ares in the *Wonder Woman* movie, the White Witch in *The Lion, the Witch and the Wardrobe*, Voldemort in Harry Potter, that type of thing. All of those stories have a message within them that you can have too much power. The media would apparently like us to believe that power is dangerous, and perhaps to be avoided unless you are one of the special, gifted few (given magical powers at birth; Jesus disguised as a lion; an actual god). Even then, the gifted ones often experience a terrible consequence because of their power: I refer you to Spiderman's tragic love life, Black Widow's enforced hysterectomy and stolen childhood and the melting of the witch in *The Wizard of Oz*.

This, quite frankly, is bollocks.

As I said, there are different types of power, and becoming em-powered (deliberate spelling) is what we can achieve through healing. We do not have to be specially gifted to become empowered – we don't need to be born with a special destiny or a birthmark in the shape of a pentagram. Empowerment and healing are available to all, and can never go wrong.

In the wonderful book *Dreaming the Dark*, the author, Starhawk, reminds us that the spiritual is always political. She describes two types of power: the difference of *power-over* and *power-from-within*. To me, this is a crucial and important difference. Power-over is what happens when humans are run by fear. *If we don't do this, something terrible will happen! Therefore, to protect ourselves, we must overpower the group we believe to be at fault here!* This is a dangerous power. The desire to overpower others can never lead to anything good.

Power-from-within is the power that happens when humans come from a centred place of being. We do not need to overpower anyone else. We can be still and connected to all-that-is because we are without fear. And that is something we can never have enough of. Nothing bad can ever happen from too much empowerment.

I think the thing to say here is that being empowered in life is not necessarily a peaceful experience. Look at Jesus. Look at the many people who are bravely embodying their truth, walking the walk, talking the talk. Millions might love them, but millions might also hate them, too. Being deeply empowered, being deeply connected to your vision and mission in life is not necessarily palatable to others, either because they disagree with you, or they are threatened by your fearless stance. This is another fear that we all have: not being liked. Ideally, everyone would love us, and we'd be wildly popular. Fear wants everyone to like us because it doesn't want us to be expelled from the tent where we might die in the wilderness.

Pffft. Sounds exhausting, though, doesn't it? All that people-pleasing. Fortunately, we now live in a world where there isn't just one campfire, one hut where everyone has to coexist and one source of food.

Healing and power are deeply, inevitably interlinked in an infinite relationship. Think of the lemniscate, the figure eight on its side, a symbol of infinity used in cultures across the world. In mythology, the Greek god Hermes' symbol is the caduceus, the two snakes crisscrossing a wand. The snakes make a repeating figure-of-eight pattern going up the rod, which looks very like the DNA helix. In my interpretation of the symbol, healing is one side of the lemniscate loop, and power is the other. The combination of the two snakes in the image, constantly crisscrossing each other, are (in my view) what make true magic and enlightenment: acknowledging and standing within the flow of creation and destruction, yin and yang, dark and light. Hermes is associated with the planet Mercury (the wings at the top of the caduceus represent his speed and reputation as the messenger of the gods), and Mercury rules, among other things, magic. To me that says that transformation – magic and enlightenment – is only to be gained by healing. If you imagine the rod part of the caduceus symbol and imagine Earth at the bottom and God at the top (simplistic, I know), then the snakes are how the human soul reaches God, enlightenment or Nirvana – whatever you want to call it. You cannot just magic your way up the rod. You've got to heal as well to get to the top.

To me, this is really important. To be power-full, to be empowered, we have to heal. And the more we heal (and everyone needs it, regardless of what you think you have in that noggin) the more powerful we become in manifesting our true desires because we aren't getting in our own way anymore with all our inherited wounds, our trauma, our learned bad patterns, and all the rest. The more we heal, the more powerful we feel to make good changes in our lives. For example, someone might realize that:

- I've left my poverty consciousness behind, therefore I can feel confident about setting up my own consultancy business.
- I've moved on from letting my fear of love run my romantic life, so now I can attract a good partner into my life and know how to be open to them.
- I've let go of my childhood trauma and invested lots of love in my inner child, and I now feel happier and more joyful, and less resentful.

And, ergo, these good choices we are now empowered to make, create more ripples of satisfaction in our lives, leading us to move on to healing other things in our lives and in the wider world.

I firmly believe, therefore, that we all have the responsibility to self-heal, to transmute our part of whatever ancestral, generational and historic traumas we have a connection to, before we can properly start to manifest our wishes in this material world. Healing is an essential part of the work; we can't expect to vision-board our way to bliss without opening up that dark cupboard and looking at what's inside, ready to sabotage us at the first snip of the scissors on the glossy magazine. Yet, once we've done that (in whatever way we find best; I've tried a few), our visions for the future can much more easily jump into being.

Just like witchcraft.

Interview with Ana, past life regression therapist

Could you describe what past life regression is?

First, I should say that hypnosis, which is the technique used in past life regression, is an extremely relaxed state in which we are able to access parts of our mind or brain that we would find difficult to access otherwise. The hypnotic state is between the dream and waking state, and hypnosis allows us to access the unconscious part of the brain where we find emotions, imagination and memory. We can access this place through meditation or something like shamanic journeying, but it's all the same thing, and in that state, we can recall things that we might not otherwise be able to recall.

When I go into past life regression with a client it's usually because they have a trauma that is manifesting in this life that they can't clear by addressing the events in this life alone. When we go to the past life, I regress the client back to their childhood in a hypnosis session, but focus only on happy memories, as we don't want to get stuck in their trauma from this life. Then we go back into the womb, and then we go to the past lives. There are stages that we go through to get there.

It might take one session or many sessions to resolve a past life issue; it very much depends on the individual and how quickly they can attain the level of relaxation that will allow them to go there, and whether the issue is rooted in more than one lifetime. With some clients, we've started off focusing on something in this life and then they've spontaneously started talking about a past life.

Clients will typically remember what happens when they've been under hypnosis, sometimes in detail, and sometimes not so much detail. Again, it's a highly individual experience, different every time.

Why do you do past life regression with clients?

Past life regression is always done to release trauma and not just out of curiosity. I would never do this just for fun; it's serious and, I would say, sacred work, and always for the purpose of healing. Clients might come to me with a phobia or a chronic condition and they want to know where it's coming from. Perhaps they've exhausted all other ways to tackle the problem – and then the adventure begins. I think of it as a journey with each client, a journey of the soul that might have become stuck in trauma in the past.

Is it something everyone would benefit from, or perhaps it's not for everyone?

I believe everyone does have past life trauma. In theory everyone would benefit from past life regression therapy, but that doesn't mean it's necessary for everybody.

I might add here that I'm also an astrologer as well as a clinical hypnotherapist and past life regression therapist. In my experience, many of the issues that we have experienced in past lives are echoed in this one. So, we get the chance to resolve those issues in this life: I believe we deliberately come into this life with chosen issues to deal with here, and we have set up a series of experiences that will require us to address those traumas or issues from a previous life.

This can involve dealing with those issues purely from this life's perspective, and there's no need to go back into past lives to do that. For example, if you have an issue with your mother in this life, there is a strong possibility that these issues have been there in previous lives, but that doesn't mean that we have to revisit those previous lives. We might be able to resolve that mother issue in this life by working through it in the here and now. However, there are times when that's not enough. So for someone who had a life in World War Two and ended up in a concentration camp, they may have an intense fear of some situations in this life, and in that case, because of the severity and specificity of that experience, we would probably need to do a past life regression.

What's your view about the idea that when people remember past lives, they always seem to have been famous people?
What that's revealing is ignorance, I would say. If people bothered to read the literature that's out there, they would discover that almost no one goes back to a life in which they were famous. It's a popular misconception and a cliché that tends to be bandied about by people who don't know much about the subject!

How did you come to past life regression yourself?
It was a long journey! I first came across the idea from reading some novels when I was younger. Then my partner introduced me to the concept and the research. I was intrigued, and it changed my world view altogether! I was studying astrology at the time and so my understanding of past lives began to evolve along with that. But it wasn't until I trained to be a hypnotherapist that I started working with it.

I started hypnotherapy because, as an astrologer, I realized that doing people's birth charts highlighted issues that they hadn't been able to solve. People may have had conventional therapy but it hadn't helped, and I knew that hypnotherapy would help them because it allowed for that heightened sense of connection to memory through that extreme relaxed state, where you could go back to the beginning of a problem and address it there.

The idea with hypnosis – which is proven – is that we learn best and change when we are both conscious and unconscious at the same time. We are aware of what's happening, but in an extremely relaxed state. And then we can make connections between things that hadn't occurred to us before. There is a plasticity to the brain in this state that means we can make changes much more effectively than when we are awake.

Once I became a hypnotherapist it seemed natural to explore past life regression because it was already part of my understanding, and now I had the tools to do it. I studied with the Michael Newton Institute and then went on to study techniques for "Life Between Life" work.

What's "Life Between Life" work?

When we pass over we aren't instantly incarnate in another body, so there is an inbetween state, and "Life Between Life" work is about accessing memories from the time spent in that place.

Can you tell me about a meaningful healing experience you've had with past life regression?

I haven't done a lot of past life regression myself, but I have had spontaneous memories of past lives which tend to be triggered by something in the same way that memories in this life are triggered.

I was watching a TV show one day about buying properties abroad, and they were in the South of France – the Languedoc area in particular – and they went to Carcassonne – a very old, medieval city. When I saw it, I started to sob, because I knew it was home, and I desperately had the sense that I wanted to go home to see it. I'd never been there in this life.

The interesting thing was that for years I'd had nightmares of a particular kind and had my suspicions that something very brutal had happened to me in a past life. And when I saw Carcassonne, I knew it was linked to that place.

When I researched the area, I learned that it was one of the cities populated by the Cathars at one time, a Christian group that was persecuted by the Catholic Church to the degree that Carcassonne saw a brutal genocide of the Cathars. And that was what I was feeling: a knowledge that I had been there and something terrible had happened to me then.

Later, I visited Carcassonne and when I got to the city wall I felt such a huge fear. I didn't want to go in. When I did go in, there were parts of the city that felt very familiar to me. When I went into the church, I couldn't stay for more than a couple of minutes. I just had to get out; I just had a terrible feeling. I learned afterwards that when the city had been attacked, the people of Carcassonne had taken refuge in the church, and the church had been burned down with them in it.

How has past life regression changed your life?
An understanding of the process of reincarnation and the life between life period has cemented my understanding that life continues, and there is a meaning to what happens to us. It isn't random. We don't always have the big picture, so sometimes it's hard to understand the pain we're going through. But there's always a reason, and it's always with the intention that our soul will grow from the experience. It's an experience that, a long time ago and in another dimension, we decided that we needed to have, no matter how hard it is for us to understand.

When you have that understanding, it begins to make sense of life.

CHAPTER 6

REMEMBERING THE "MAGICAL ME" AND WITCHCRAFT AS AN EMPOWERING FORCE

As a teenager in the 90s, I discovered the movie *The Craft*, listened obsessively to grunge rock geniuses Nirvana and feminist riot grrrl bands like Bikini Kill, and decided I was going to be a witch. Finally, something that didn't require A Levels.[1]

Modern witchcraft had experienced a huge moment of expansion in the 90s with a raft of new books published on the subject by Llewellyn in the US, and modern witches like Janet and Stewart Farrar in the UK publishing a series of guides to modern witchcraft. These books introduced me to what it was like to work magic in a coven, to psychic self-defence and the concept of the wheel of the year, celebrating the old pagan festivals as a means of connecting oneself to the natural rhythms of the earth.[2] The first book I ever read on the subject was Janet

---

[1] I'm joking, and I did do my A Levels. Stay in school, kids!

[2] In fact, modern witchcraft – or Wicca, as it was best known then – had been around since Gerald Gardner wrote his exposé of what he called "the witch cult" in his book *Witchcraft Today* in 1954. According to Gardner and other historians such as Ronald Hutton, witches had been doing their thing for a long time before that, too.

and Stewart Farrar's *What Witches Do*,[3] and it began a lifelong passion for magic.

Fast-forward to a few years after my son was born, and I'd maintained my general witchy interests for some time. In between work, parenting, writing and trying to maintain some kind of social life, I would do rituals in my garden at night, read books about goddesses, read the tarot for myself and others and learn new things when I could.

I'd also stayed in contact with a friend, Laura, whom I'd met on a tarot course in the same year I'd discovered reiki. Laura was now a professional tarot reader and witch and we had both become interested in one particular Celtic goddess, the Morrigan. I'd found myself writing about the Morrigan as well as the Celtic gods Lugh and Brighid in a fictional trilogy I was working on at the time.

Brighid (closely related to St Bridget in the Catholic tradition) is a goddess of fire, transformation, healing and art, among other things. As a fire goddess she rules hearth and home and is also responsible for our creative fire and inspiration. Lugh is a sun god, a warrior and a king, connected with the harvest. In fact, the pagan harvest festival of Lughnasadh (also known as Lammas) is named after him.

The Morrigan is, at first glance, terrifying. Part of the deep mythology of the Celtic tradition told in old texts such as the 12th-century *Lebor Gabála Érenn* (The Book of the Taking of Ireland) and the *Cath Maige Tuired* (The Battle of Magh Tuireadh), she is a goddess of war, death, sexuality and the underworld; of fairyland and magic; and a protector of women and the land. She is often depicted dressed in black, accompanied by crows and ravens, and was said to give soldiers visions of washing their own bloody armour if they were about to die on the battlefield. She was also said to fly like a crow

---

[3] There are, of course, hundreds of excellent books about witchcraft, and I've included a list of my recommendations at the end of this book, with plenty for beginners.

above battle, terrifying one side of the battle and inspiring confidence and hope in the other.

People often don't expect witchcraft to involve gods, but one's connection to archetypes of gods and goddesses is a key element for many. Although not all, it has to be said: many modern witches may consider their focus to be more on spirit[4] than on gods, and others again don't believe in gods at all. Modern witchcraft is a very broad, anarchic and decentralized church.

Yet, I think, for many of us – especially those of us brought up with patriarchal religions – one of the many appeals of a witchcraft practice is its embracing of goddesses. As a girl, as a young person, as a woman, it is intensely empowering to have an all-powerful goddess to relate to, to pray to, to learn stories about. The study of witchcraft can often become the study of other religions, both contemporary and ancient. Gods from all manner of different religions and practices are popular in witchcraft, from the ancient Greek, Norse, Roman and Egyptian pantheons to the Celtic, old British or Hindu gods and the Native American traditions. In some modern practices, emphasis is even on working with our modern "gods" of celebrity, cybercurrency, fashion and other currents of energy.[5]

Another appeal of witchcraft is its emphasis on one's direct contact with the gods or spirits: there's no priest, rabbi or vicar needed to intercede on your behalf. Your relationship with the gods is your own, and witchcraft traditionally prioritizes practices such as tarot, astrology and the development of psychic

---

[4] i.e. the spirits of the dead, ancestors, natural spirits belonging to the classic four elements (in Wicca, earth spirits are gnomes, air spirits are sylphs, water spirits are undines and fire spirits are salamanders), animal spirits, or the various leagues of angels in the angelic or ceremonial magic traditions. In other cultures, of course, beliefs and practices are varied again, from the orishas and loa of Yoruba, Haitian and other African cultures to the huldufólk in Iceland and many more. There is much crossover in different cultures between what is considered spirit and what is considered a god.

[5] This kind of modern approach comes, I think in part, from a tradition called chaos magic, which is well worth investigating but which I don't have the space to explain here!

abilities as a means to better connect with the gods, spirits and the spiritual teachers in other realms.

Third, I think a big appeal is its emphasis on working collaboratively with nature. Nowadays, people are more aware of things like which phase of the moon we're in, when the next Mercury retrograde is and what the names of the plants are that grow in their local area. It seems to me that people have a deep need to reconnect to nature in these days of hyperconnectivity and living online: I see more and more courses teaching people how to forage, grow food and how to calibrate their lives to the natural cycles of the year. More people are also adopting old traditions (in the UK, these are some examples) like wassailing[6] and setting places at the dinner table for dead relatives at Samhain (the Celtic festival for the dead, held on 31 October – now known as Halloween).

Witchcraft encourages you to become aware of nature around you, of natural places of power you can visit to recharge, to meditate, even to do magical work and spells. It encourages you to connect with the elemental powers and to ask for their help. It teaches you that gods and goddesses often represent different elements of nature, and that by connecting with the gods you are also connecting to that element of nature in your own psyche. In connecting with moon goddesses, you are connecting to feeling the flux of your own energies, both physical, mental and emotional, as well as your dream world. In connecting with the goddess Brighid, you can examine your creativity and passion.

Connecting to the Morrigan – a hardcore goddess of death, war and our journeys through the underworld – means that you are probably *going through some shit*.[7]

For some reason, as I was writing about the Morrigan in my novel, I started to come across other women who were also interested in this goddess, so much so that when Laura invited me

---

[6] Venerating your apple trees so they keep giving you apples. Involves much cider drinking.

[7] But also that you will come out the other side, healed and renewed. Phew!

to a weekend Morrigan retreat, I said yes. When you have young children, the prospect of getting away for a weekend on your own to do anything is pretty appealing, never mind the prospect of being with other women in Glastonbury doing witchy things. I bought a new black velour tracksuit for the occasion (in my defence, the dress code read "comfortable") and off I went.

The first thing I realized when I arrived was that, no matter how magical you think you are, fitting 12 middle-aged women into a one-bedroom house is a logistical nightmare. Where does everyone sleep? It's a bit like that joke: how do you get four elephants into a Mini? (Two in the front, two in the back, of course.) I had the advantage – I got to share Laura's room – but otherwise, people were lined up on sinking airbeds in the lounge, in a tent in the garden and one of us was making the best of it in a sleeping bag in an airing cupboard. Also, 12 women, one bathroom, plus a vegetarian menu for the weekend. Hmmm.

We began by doing a getting-to-know-you circle in the lounge,[8] and then went out for a walk to explore the mythic land around Glastonbury. One of my abiding memories of this weekend is that, as we walked through the lush, dense Somerset forest, we found a swing attached to a tree (thankfully, a sturdy one) and all took turns swinging madly on it for half an hour or more. Goodness knows what any passing dog walker would have made of us.

Atop a wide, grassy hill, Laura led us in a guided visualization as we lay on our backs under the afternoon sun, and we connected with the Morrigan in her earth goddess aspect as well as visiting her under the hill in her faery realm, asking what advice she had for us. Listening to the beat of the drum as Laura guided us into the otherworld was a beautiful and visionary experience.

That night, we held a circle in the tent in the garden. Laura and the two other witches in charge of the weekend created a

---

[8] There was nothing particularly witchy about this. If you've ever attended any sort of course or training event, it's just that cringeworthy bit at the beginning where you have to introduce yourself and say what you hope to get out of the course.

sacred space in the tent with prayer, incense and some traditional circle-casting methods: tracing a circle around your space with the four elements in turn and asking the elemental powers to be with you in protection and to lend their power to you. One by one, we were "smudged" with sage smoke by Sian as we filed into the circular tent.

Inside, we all sat around the edge and began by making personal offerings to the Morrigan, which we'd been asked to do before attending. As a natural teacher's pet, homework is something I have always prided myself on going the extra mile with, and so I'd prepared a collaged mini altar to the Morrigan from half an apple box and a wealth of cut-out pictures, photos, text and crow feathers. I placed mine in the centre of the circle along with the gifts from the other attendees, which were all different and equally beautiful and personal to their makers. Some people explained what they'd brought; some people just quietly placed their offerings.

I didn't quite know what to expect from the circle. Were we going to do some spellwork? Were we going to chant? What would happen next? I'd done quite a lot of witchy activities on my own, including casting circles and spells, and honouring the passing seasons at the times of the festivals, but I hadn't worked much with other people at that point. Would we all get naked? Was that why comfortable (and, ergo, easily removable) clothes had been specified?

I'm going to manage your expectations of a sex orgy right now and tell you that no one got naked, not least because it was October in England and it was fricking freezing sitting on the hard ground – and it would have been pretty irrelevant to our aims for the evening anyway. Instead, we did something perhaps even more exposing and vulnerable: we shared our real reasons for coming to the Morrigan, and some of those were difficult to hear.

I won't go into details here, as what was shared was private and personal for the women involved. What I will say is that I'm proud to have helped hold the space for those women to share their sometimes-difficult truth. In retrospect, I realized what we were doing was holding a red tent,[9] an old tradition for women to come together and share their stories in a safe space. As a warlike protectress of women, the Morrigan is a good goddess to listen to our painful experiences. I shared my feelings about being a mother, and how hard I'd found it for those first few years.

From the start, my son's arrival into the world had been difficult. Was it an unhealed mother wound on my part that made it so hard? Perhaps. Either way, almost as soon as my pregnancy began, I developed crippling sciatica that meant it was difficult to walk around or do anything. If you've never experienced sciatica, then CONGRATULATIONS, because it is godawful. In fact, I recall that my mum also suffered with it when I was at secondary school. There were days I'd leave for school with her draped over the washing basket on her hands and knees because it was the only way she could reduce the pain – and I'd return to find her still there. With sciatica, what happens is that the sciatic nerve that runs from your lower back down to your feet is caught or compressed in some way, resulting in extreme pain and difficulty getting around. Apparently, it's more likely in pregnancy because everything in your body, especially in the lower body, is changing and moving around and whatnot.

The doctor breezily dismissed my EXTREME PAIN (as doctors are wont to do with women, I find) and told me that it would likely ease up in a few weeks.

It did not.

I was in fact in debilitating pain throughout my pregnancy (as well as "morning" sickness, AKA all-day-long nausea, fun!) and well into the second year of my son's life, when I finally started doing yoga and strengthened my core. I'd seen osteopaths throughout the two years as well, who were very helpful, but it

---

[9]   You can read Anita Diamant's novel of the same name to get an idea. Diamant writes about biblical times where the Jewish women in the novel would retreat to a particular tent during menstruation or after childbirth to recover, menstruate, and be cared for by the other women, often exchanging stories to pass the time and support each other. I actually used this idea of a (more inclusive) sharing space for people identifying as women in my novel *The Book of Babalon*.

was the yoga – and specifically plank exercises – that got rid of it. I mean, I generally dislike exercise, and planks (where you are basically in a stationary press-up with your arms straight – or balanced on your forearms. You can also side plank for extra fun) are particularly non-pleasurable. HOWEVER, it did strengthen my back and stomach muscles enough (I guess) for them to hold my nerves where they should be, and for me to stand up straighter and be free from pain.

THANK. GOD.

I cannot express to you how painful sciatica is, but imagine it when you also have a heavy, wriggly baby who wants to be carried all day long. It was a living nightmare. I remember one week it was so bad that my friend who was visiting had to put my son into and take him out of his cot for me because I just couldn't bend. It was completely impossible.

So, that had been going on for me. But that's not even approaching what else had happened.

When it came time for my son to be born, my contractions began in a normal way. We went to the hospital to get checked out. Everything seemed to be going to plan from my point of view: my waters had broken and I had a TENS machine which was helping with the contraction pain pretty well. I probably had the normal amount of trepidation about the birth but, also, at that point you're just so keen to move on from being heavily pregnant that you want it all to happen already. If you're reading this and you've delivered a baby, you know this.

Yet, when the nurses in the maternity ward examined me, they discovered that my son was lying transverse (diagonally) in my uterus, completely the wrong way around, and there was no way that he could be born naturally. Therefore, I had to have an emergency caesarean section, like, IMMEDIATELY. I had been in labour for maybe eight to ten hours at this point.

This was really scary for me. I was already pretty phobic about hospitals from my experiences with my mum, and I'd made it this far in life without any major surgery, but now I had to have it WHILE BEING AWAKE, and I had to have it RIGHT

NOW as my son was increasingly at risk. I started to panic. Perhaps half an hour after that, I was wheeled into the operating theatre where a nurse who looked like a rugby player held up a massive syringe in his huge hands and proceeded to inject it into my spine, despite the fact that I was halfway through a panic attack at the time. In his defence, he wasn't being insensitive to my feelings on purpose; it was just more the fact that, when things are going south in childbirth, there isn't really time to take feelings into account.

Twenty minutes later, my son was held up before my eyes. He took a while to cry, and I think there was some anxiety that he wouldn't breathe. I remember lying there as the nurses took him away to be weighed and tested and whatever else they do to newborn babies, while the other doctors started stitching me up and my deathly white husband tried valiantly to hold on to his breakfast, listening in the silence for our new baby's cry, waiting as the seconds stretched on and on.

Finally, he cried. Arguably, he didn't stop crying after that for a good two years.

We were both pretty traumatized by the birth, I think. However, after spending two days in hospital we were released, and I returned home severely exhausted and having undergone major surgery, and was now expected to look after a newborn.

As an aside here, I really don't think we have it quite right as a culture when it comes to how we look after new mothers. How can it be kind and fair to leave a new mother essentially to her own devices after something as potentially traumatic, painful and debilitating as childbirth? Yes, some women have a good birth and then a great support network in place to look after them and the baby afterwards. But many women also don't. What about them?

Naively, I had supposed that after having a baby, I'd be up and about in a day or two, breezily breastfeeding while stacking the dishwasher; perhaps I'd pop out for a coffee with the baby sleeping quietly, and of course I'd have time to brush my teeth and get dressed every day.

Of course I would. Who doesn't brush their teeth every day? New mothers, that's who.

Ten days after my son was born, he developed a funny rash, mostly on his face. Now, I didn't know that it was funny, because I'd never had a baby before, but when the health visitor came round, she told me she didn't like the look of it, and sent me and my son in to A&E.

Imagine, if you will, being ten days post emergency C-section, hardly able to stand, breastfeeding, sleep-deprived and alone (my husband had just gone back to work), and facing a trip to A&E with the baby you still call "the baby" because it hasn't quite sunk in yet that they are a real actual person, and that you are a hundred per cent responsible for them.

In a panic, I phoned my dad, who came over and drove me to the hospital.[10]

At the hospital, I was convinced that the health visitor had it wrong. Babies get rashes; it's not a big deal. I thought she was over-reacting. I really resented having to come to A&E because I still hated hospitals.

However, when the doctors examined my new baby, their frowns didn't disappear.

A very kind young paediatric doctor sat down with my husband (who had driven back from work in a panic) and me. "Okay, what we think is that this rash is herpes. But there is a risk that this might lead to meningitis, so we're going to need to keep you here."[11]

---

[10] I was not allowed to drive for six weeks after the C-section.

11 Herpes meningoencephalitis is the name of the condition the doctors were worried about. The meninges are the layers of thin tissue that cover your brain. If these tissues become infected, it's called meningitis. When your brain becomes inflamed or infected, the problem is called encephalitis. If both the meninges and the brain are infected, the condition is called meningoencephalitis.

Encephalitis involving herpes is a medical emergency that needs to be promptly diagnosed and treated. It is often fatal when left untreated. Encephalitis is caused by the herpes simplex virus. Most are caused by herpes simplex virus type 1 (HSV1), the virus that also causes cold sores. It can also be caused by herpes simplex virus type 2 (HSV2), which can be spread from mother to baby during childbirth.

Meningitis is one of the words that no parent ever wants to hear. It's a condition where the protective membranes that surround the brain and spinal cord get infected, which can lead to blood poisoning and even death. My cousin's baby boy died from meningitis, and it is a terrifying, awful thing that no one should have to experience. Viruses such as mumps, herpes and tummy bugs can all cause it, as can bacteria such as the Hib (Haemophilus influenzae type b) and pneumonia bacteria. Luckily, in the UK we have an excellent vaccination programme that includes mumps, Hib and pneumonia (I will always be grateful for the existence of vaccination, and you can bet I took my son in as soon as I could to have him vaccinated at three months and six months old), but there's no herpes vaccine.

"How long?" I asked, my heart in my mouth.

"Two weeks," the doctor replied. "We'll be giving your son antiviral drugs every eight hours, intravenously. So, you can come and go in between sessions, if you want, but you have to be here every eight hours, regardless."

Two weeks.

I couldn't drive because of the caesarean. My husband at the time couldn't drive and was at work. So it looked like my son and I were stuck there.

Worse was the process that led to a proper diagnosis: they had to do a lumbar puncture on my ten-day-old baby to test his spinal fluid for meningitis. This means that the doctor sticks a needle into the baby's spine, while having to hold them still, because if they damage the spinal cord then they could paralyse your baby.

I remember standing outside the doors of the paediatric A&E sobbing my heart out with my husband as the doctors performed the lumbar puncture. It was something they recommended we weren't present for, knowing that it would be too traumatic to watch.

I felt like a failure. I had failed my baby. Other new mothers were out, taking walks in the park, having picnics, being looked after by their families. I had failed to look after him well enough and now he was being jabbed with syringes and handed around like a tiny test subject.

Almost as bad as the lumbar puncture was watching as the nurses tried to get an IV into my son's tiny little arm. The thing with babies is that they wriggle a lot, and they have tiny veins. Plus, I learned pretty quickly, they don't like having an IV. My son ripped his out on countless occasions, only to have to have it put back in. This whole process was heartbreaking.

So, there we were, in a hospital room (fortunately, we were given one on our own), having an hour's antiviral infusion every eight hours and trying to manage being normal the rest of the time. I worked out that if I breastfed my son while he had his infusion, that would make him calm enough not to twist the IV around, so after a few shaky days we fell into a kind of routine.

I tried to sleep in the times between the infusions – and tried to get him to sleep – but, as we all know, hospitals are loud, busy places with people constantly charging into your room to do one thing or another. We also seemed popular with the student doctors who kept coming in to ask questions. I kept it together: I was polite and helpful and as good-humoured as I could be, but really, I just wanted to scream at everyone, tell them to fuck off and give us some peace and quiet.

Unsurprisingly, my son wasn't the most placid of babies during this experience, and spent most of the two weeks screaming the hospital down. He slept only by lying on my chest and had to be on me at all times or he'd go postal. Even going to the toilet required me to buzz a nurse who would come in and watch him while I dashed to the toilet down the hall, listening to him cry. Showering was a distant dream. I don't think I showered for the first eight days I was in hospital, that time around.

I remember one night in particular, walking him up and down in that little room we had, up and down, my abdomen killing me, sweating because it was a June heatwave and the hospital was even hotter inside than outside. I couldn't get him to stop crying. My whole life had reduced to one small room. No one offered to come and take us out for a few hours, and even if we could have left, I don't think we would have been great company. All we had was each other and the visitors we had here and there: my husband for a couple of hours in the evening after work, my dad and a few friends who made the trip.

It was a dark, dark two weeks for me. I had now not slept for more than three weeks, I'd barely eaten, and my stress levels were through the roof. There's also something intensely stressful (to me, anyway) about having a baby on your body AT ALL TIMES. Your body is not your own at this time. If my son wasn't breastfeeding, he was sleeping on me or needing to be walked up and down or held to be pacified. Add to all this your own body recovering from major surgery.

Finally, after two weeks of antiviral treatment, we were allowed to leave. As you can imagine, I was *very* glad to get back home. I remember looking in amazement at how green the garden was. How colourful my house was with its lovely fabrics.

After this rough start to motherhood, I needed a support network (and all parents need support, in fact, because it is a bloody difficult job). Over time, I made friends with other new parents and asked advice from my existing parent friends, which has always been invaluable. But one thing I also needed was to sit in a circle with other women and tell my story. It wouldn't be for everyone, but for me the ritualized setting helped. It felt good to have a sense of occasion about it all, and to also relate my experience back to a goddess who is a protector of women. The Morrigan, as a warrior, reminded me of my own capacity to fight, to be strong, to do what I had to do in times of survival. I suppose it's like having a focus for your experience, a symbol and a story that can help you process what you have endured.

Connecting with the Morrigan in this setting, with other women, made me feel stronger. The power of a community — being present to witness the stories of others in the circle, and knowing that your story is heard – was profound for my healing.

Interview with Laura Daligan – witch

Can you explain what your witchcraft looks like? What are your main principles and beliefs, in a nutshell?

My witchcraft is entwined into my everyday life: there's so much I do with my daily work which is part of my witchcraft and spiritual path. I'm a tarot reader and an artist, and in my art I often do journeys or meditations to gods or goddesses or animal spirits. So for me, witchcraft isn't usually so much a spell to attain something, it's more about connection. I'm someone who likes to quest, to meet and understand the gods and get to know them.

That said, I do rituals, I celebrate the seasons and the pagan festivals of the year, I work with the moon cycles – new moon, full moon and banishing on the dark moon. I have an altar where I light a candle every day, light some incense and have that daily connection to the divine. So it's these little practices that keep my magical life on track.

I have an animistic belief that the divine flows through everything. There's no separate part of my life that's witchcraft; it permeates everything I do. Even the washing up! Well, maybe not that …

How does healing fit into your experience of witchcraft?

When I worked in a coven and someone needed healing, we'd work together to focus our energy and make that the focus of our ritual and bring that intent into manifestation. I remember once we worked for the intention for one of the girls to get pregnant, but I excluded myself from that ritual, just in case the energy mistook me for a wannabe mother! I was like, *No, not me!* I have to say it's really nice to work with a group of other like-minded people when you want to manifest healing.

Now I'm working as a solitary witch, it's more about knowing about what energy is best to work with at certain times for healing. So at the dark moon I do a lot of cleansing and salt baths to clear my energy field, and at Beltane (1 May) I call in love and abundance for emotional healing.

I also work with shamanic healing, so that's the practice of a kind of imaginative journeying to a drum beat into the upper or lower worlds, as they're called. The upper world contains spirit guides or different natural psychic landscapes and the lower worlds also contain animal spirits. I journey to find the healing or to find guidance or a spirit guide that will help with the problem. That's a really powerful and interesting way of working with healing too.

Is witchcraft itself a healing and empowering experience? How?

It's a shame in so many ways that there isn't a continuous tradition of witchcraft in our culture, because of the inherent empowerment that it brings. But when you do discover it, the power of it and that "coming home" feeling many people get when connecting to witchcraft, the healing power of that connection is so massive in itself.

I think when you say you are a witch or you work with witchcraft, you're saying, *I have power. I am aligned with power, and I'm someone that knows myself,* or I'm working on myself anyway. In that way it's a very powerful and empowering and healing statement because there's so much around us that takes that power away. Telling us we have to be small, or fit into boxes. When we say *I'm a witch,* it's very outside the box! Maybe less so now than when I first said it twenty years ago, but it's still very outside what's known in society. But as soon as we make that connection to the world around us, we realize that we are powerful and we don't need a middle man to make that connection to power for us. Nature is powerful and alive, and you really feel that when you start to work with witchcraft. And when I say "nature" I also mean the deities that typify those natural forces in the universe.

How did you come to witchcraft in the first place?

I think initially it was through the music and art I liked – a lot of the musicians I liked were quite interested in the occult.

When I was a teenager I bought books on Wicca, like Vivianne Crowley's book *Wicca*, which is a good foundation text. But I wasn't ready then, and you do really need to be ready to do the work and all it entails. Then when I was twenty-two and living in London I came across a tarot course, and I just knew it was for me. On that course we ended up going to an open pagan ritual because it was in the same building on the same day. So the tarot helped me open up my awareness and intuition but walking into that room with the incense and the chanting and the ritual elements, I just knew that I was home in a very deep soul way. That's when I started walking that path.

So can you tell me one particular experience in your personal healing journey that was really meaningful in some way?
When I did my second-degree initiation for the coven, I had to sit out all night in nature, which I did on Hampstead Heath in London. The idea in the second degree is that it's all about facing your shadow, and having the strength and will to go out there and face your demons, as it were, and put yourself in the hands of nature in quite a vulnerable way. And then also experience the dawn at the end of it. I think the fact that people are expecting you to do it as a very formal part of your coven work means that it makes you actually sit it out for the whole night. Otherwise, if it was just something you were doing for yourself, you'd probably head off home after a few hours! It's about pushing through your boundaries and testing yourself as a kind of endurance.

On one hand it was terrifying because I thought of every horror movie I'd ever seen, and there I was, sitting in the dark all night. But then when the sun rose and I walked out into the day, that was so transformational. You can imagine that sitting out all night on Hampstead Heath was a kind of dark night of the soul experience – it was hard to go through, and uncomfortable, and I was at the mercy of the elements, which we're really not used to in this day and age! But I would say it's an amazing experience to put yourself at the mercy of the elements in that way, as long as it's safe, or you're as safe as you can be. Coming out of that dark night, every sense is heightened, and I did feel amazing, witnessing that daily return of the light. And it happens every day, yet usually we're asleep and unaware of it. I have to say I think I frightened some joggers as I emerged from the bushes in the early hours!

How has witchcraft changed your life?
It's hard to say because it's so huge – it's changed my career, my friendships, my personal life. My YouTube channel is LauraRedWitch and that's how people know me! In a more profound way, it's changed the way I connect with the gods and nature, about understanding that there is truth embedded in mythology and they aren't just stories. It's part of the thread of my life, and it's hard to imagine what came before. I think witchcraft makes you live in the here and now, and it's a way of understanding if not what you're here for, then what you can do while you are here.

CHAPTER 7

MOOING WITH YOUR EYES CLOSED: MOTHERHOOD AND SHAMANIC JOURNEYING

It was a summer Saturday in a community centre in southwest London, and I was stamping my hooves and mooing forcefully, trying to disconnect from my natural British reserve that was convincing me that channelling the spirit of a cow was a completely ridiculous thing to be doing.

Still, at least I wasn't alone. It wasn't like the time I took a "kung fu with swords" class and everyone had to demonstrate the moves individually, in front of the class. That was pure hell (and, no doubt, punishment from the gods of kung fu, who knew I was only at the class to impress a boy I liked. Unfortunately, when formulating this foolproof seduction plan, I didn't factor in my ineptitude for martial arts and sports of any kind. Literally none of you will be surprised to learn that I never got to be that guy's girlfriend, which was a great shame, because he was insanely hot). Today, there were around 30 of us in the school hall, and we were ALL ridiculous. In a way, that was quite encouraging.

It is my conclusion that classical shamanism (which is what we were learning) is a very beautiful, powerful, sacred collection of practices which look ridiculous if observed by outsiders without any context.

Shamanic practices are present across many cultures.[1] The shaman is traditionally a powerful figure within a community who uses altered states of consciousness to speak to the spirits of nature, to the ancestors and the spirit world, who can travel to the human and animal or nature spirit worlds and gain power from the spirits there. She can heal others and intercede with the spirits on their behalf. She can assist people when they are dying and help lead them to the spirit worlds, and she can guide the members of her community in vision, journeying and enlightenment. Often, shamans are skilled herbalists and healers, having an intimate knowledge of and relationship with their local flora and fauna.

Shamanic traditions across the world have many similarities, but also many cultural differences. Some of the most well-known practices come from the Native American traditions (in themselves varied), South American cultures from the Andes to Chile and Argentina, from Inuit cultures, Siberia, Haiti (the practice of voudoun) and Hawaii. However, many other indigenous cultures also have traditions that involve a shaman

---

[1] The English historian Ronald Hutton noted that by the dawn of the 21st century, there were four separate definitions of the term "shaman" which appeared to be in use:
- The first of these uses the term to refer to "anybody who contacts a spirit world while in an altered state of consciousness".
- The second definition limits the term to refer to those who contact a spirit world while in an altered state of consciousness at the behest of others.
- The third definition attempts to distinguish shamans from other magico-religious specialists who are believed to contact spirits, such as mediums, witch doctors, spiritual healers or prophets, by claiming that shamans undertake some particular technique not used by the others.
- The fourth definition identified by Hutton uses "shamanism" to refer to the indigenous religions of Siberia and neighbouring parts of Asia. en.wikipedia.org/wiki/Shamanism

or priest of some kind gaining wisdom or healing for others via altered states of consciousness.

The shamanic practices that we learn in the West come from the work of anthropologist Michael Harner[2] and Mircea Eliade, and, more recently in the US and UK, Sandra Ingerman and Steven Farmer. The "modern shamanic renaissance" that occurred in the West from the 1970s onwards is based on a synthesized, or combined, version of common features from a variety of South American and Native American, Siberian and Inuit practices. Harner's rationale was that we in the West are outsiders to these shamanic practices, and not members of certain tribes. Therefore, it made sense to create a system for Westerners that would teach us the main techniques but also recognize that we live in modern Western environments and with modern lifestyles and so may be unable to replicate certain more traditional elements of ages-old practices that are particular to a certain region.[3]

Now, in more recent years, there has been understandable backlash against the idea that a group of 30 white people (note: my class was fairly diverse, but the principle remains) messing about in community centres, pretending to be cows, are "doing" shamanism right. These days, we understand that cultural appropriation is something that must be seriously considered, especially when a vulnerable culture's sacred practices have been studied, learnt and then taught to Westerners for cash without those cultures being directly mentioned, remunerated or acknowledged. That has happened, and continues to happen.

---

[2]   *The Way of the Shaman* by Michael Harner

3   One of the best books I've ever read is Malidoma Patrice Some's *Of Water and the Spirit*, which I urge you to run out and buy now, or borrow from your local library. Malidoma was raised in a shamanic tribal tradition in Burkina Faso, and then forced to become a Catholic at a nearby Jesuit school. His story is both heartbreaking – due to being forced to abandon his culture and language – but the experiences he writes of when he returns to his tribe are among the most magical things you will ever read, specifically about shamanic magical practices.

However, what I would say is that I was very grateful and glad to learn from skilled instructors who had, in their turn, learnt from respectful teachers – all of whom were knowledgeable about the origins of the different traditions they had received, and were passionate about passing on that wisdom to us for little cost and, importantly, with great respect for the cultures from which they were originally learnt. I did a number of training courses in classical shamanism with a UK organization called The Sacred Trust[4] and, rather than being exploitative, I felt that my teachers cared deeply about imbuing us with a sense of wonder and mystery at the practices of the shamans, and explained to us many times about where what we were learning came from. They taught us how indigenous shamans worked, what they had learnt from the indigenous cultures they had worked with and how we could work respectfully with those traditions at all times. The Sacred Trust also run courses in European shamanic traditions such as the lesser-known Path of Pollen (also known as bee priestessing), an ancient tradition apparently present in the UK for many centuries,[5] as well as healing techniques based in Buddhist practice.

The introduction to shamanism taught us – among other things – a physical method of embodying animal spirits as a means of empowerment while in a trance state brought about by drumming. The idea is that you embody the animal spirit as much as possible. You are encouraged to make the movements and sounds of the animal (a cow, in my case) with eyes closed to preserve the trance. In practice, yes, it looks ridiculous from the outside: 30 snorting, neighing and growling adults twirling, pawing, rolling and stamping their way around a community centre is quite something to behold.[6]

---

4   I would highly recommend any of the courses from sacredtrust.org
5   I also highly recommend reading Simon Buxton's revealing and fascinating account of his work in this tradition in his book *The Shamanic Way of the Bee*.
6   I once worked at a drama school, and the Animal Study class was similarly hilarious to watch – and just as seriously taken part in.

I should add that the space we were in must have once been some kind of religious temple or gathering place, with a high ceiling and ornate steel columns holding up a mezzanine. The columns proved themselves a menace, because the aim of the exercise is to be fully immersed in the spirit of your chosen animal (you have been led to choose the animal in question in a shamanic journey, a kind of vision meditation) with your eyes closed. I'm amazed we didn't have an ambulance turning up, quite frankly, as there were several "ouch"es and very British "excuse me"s, both from banging into steel columns but also into each other. Anyway, the important thing was that we survived, we embodied our cows and jaguars and bees to the best of our ability, and could just about look each other in the eye afterwards.

I discovered The Sacred Trust after being recommended it by a couple of my friends. I'd become interested in shamanic journeying and healing after going for a shamanic healing session with a woman (whose name I have sadly forgotten; let's call her Betsy) at a local clinic, more out of curiosity than anything. Betsy was a woman who had discovered shamanic healing at some point in her life as a middle-aged woman living in Surrey. However, when she got out some fantastic hawk feathers and started singing, chanting and wafting sage smoke over me with them, I was hooked – especially when she told me I'd done shamanic work in another life. Who doesn't want to be a past-life shaman, right?

In fact, Betsy had invited me to a night of shamanic journeying at a scout hut (where else? My life of glamour continues) outside Godalming, and I'd gone along, taking part in my first ever shamanic journey. Like the true dilettante I am, I didn't continue with that group because it was actually quite a long drive and although the journeying was okay, the group work of entering trance with the drum while standing, and dancing with the drumbeat, was excruciatingly embarrassing. All I can say was that it was another instance of middle-class white people from the Home Counties self-consciously stomping around in a scout hut, trying to go into a trance, which somehow just seemed at odds with all the Waitrose tote bags lined up at the edge of the room.

To achieve shamanic journeying, you sit or lie down with a pillow and blanket (although proper tribal shamans often do it while dancing, chanting, stamping, etc.) and listen to someone drumming or using a rattle or other percussive instrument (remember the maracas or "shakers" at primary school?) in a very specific rhythm. This is a fast one-two-three-four-type rhythm aimed at inducing a theta brainwave, meditative state.[7] Theta waves are the state your brain finds in deep relaxation and dreaming.

When the drum starts, you imagine yourself at a place on earth you know, which may be a tree, a river, a hill or some kind of natural feature. It should be somewhere you've been and ideally that's special to you. I use a particular yew tree in a forest near to where I live that I've always felt an affinity with. Depending on what your place is, you imagine approaching it and entering it in some way, and either going up (in my case, I imagine climbing the tree and walking from its upper branches upwards) or down (I imagine entering a door in the tree trunk and sliding down a tunnel inside the tree and down into the earth). The real place you imagine yourself at is called your *axis mundi*, your earthly link or central point that connects the Upper World, the Middle World and the Lower World.

According to shamanic tradition, downwards takes you to the Lower World and upwards takes you to the Upper World. The world we live in is the Middle World (for any of you familiar with Norse mythology, you can see this same world view with the world tree Yggdrasil that stretches up to Asgard, the realm of the gods, through Midgard – our world – and down to Hel, the underworld).

---

[7] Dr Steven Farmer has a great article about the healing properties of drumming and the theta wave experience in journeying here: shamanicpractice.org/article/rhythm-drumming-and-shamanism

The Lower World in shamanic tradition is the place of animal and nature spirits. When you journey in your receptive, meditative state, you may imagine or vision forests, jungles, oceans, mountains, tundras, volcanoes – or any natural environment. For me it's like an awake dream. Usually you will see animals, insects, fish and reptiles there. These animal and nature spirits exist in and of themselves, but can also help and heal you, either by giving you healing in the Lower World or by agreeing to come back with you to the Middle World – our usual existence – as a Power Animal. A Power Animal is an animal spirit that gives you the essence of that animal energy you may be lacking or need. This could be anything from the playfulness of an otter to the strength of a lion. They do not belong to you, but stay for as long as you need them. You might have relationships with more than one Power Animal during your life, and sometimes important ones become long-lasting allies. The spirits of the Lower World are often interested in helping humans, and will lend you their energies in this way as long as they are approached respectfully and in the correct way.

One of the things I learnt on this course was how to do a Power Animal retrieval for someone else. We were partnered up in twos. I got partnered with a young, hot yoga-type guy in his 20s. He brought me back a penguin and I brought him back a very cute little crab. After we'd done the procedure, he said, "Does that mean you've given me crabs?"

LOL. Little bit of Power Animal humour for you there.

Many times you will begin your journey with the intention for an animal guide to communicate with you in the Lower World, to give you healing, insight into a problem or question or perhaps to come back with you to the Middle World as your Power Animal. Traditionally, the Lower World is the place to go to help heal your past. Or you can just go to explore. Exploring the Upper and Lower Worlds is really enjoyable, even without a set purpose in mind.

In the Upper World, tradition cites that you are more likely to find spiritual masters to help you vision your future and provide insight and guidance. The environment might look more "heavenly" or cloud like, or it might also look like places on earth, depending on your cultural background. I personally often visit a tundra-like or desert world which is spare and arid, but also peaceful. I often visit a spiritual guide there, a woman living in a small hut who looks after horses.

There are many levels to explore in the Upper World, and some people imagine going up and up from their axis mundi (the place on earth that acts as your imaginary transition point), maybe rising on clouds or being propelled by steam to different planes. It's not hierarchical in any way; it's not like the higher you go, the more spiritual you are. It's more that you'll end up where you're supposed to end up that time, wherever that is. Personally, when journeying to the Upper World, I imagine climbing the branches of my tree and then climbing up a transparent glassy staircase up and up until I find the place that feels right. Sometimes I imagine I go up in a transparent lift or escalator, if I really can't face all those steps.

So, we journey to the Upper and Lower Worlds to get answers to questions we have; to find enlightenment; to meet our spirit guides and power animals. We can also find healing in the other worlds by means of retrieving a power animal to work with us and provide an energy that might be missing in our lives, or with other methods such as soul retrieval.

The idea behind soul retrieval, in a very tiny nutshell, is that when we experience trauma of some kind, we lose a part of our soul as a result. The role of the shaman in healing that trauma is to go into the otherworlds, find that missing part of you and return it and integrate it to your soul. For more on this, Sandra Ingerman's *Soul Retrieval: Mending the Fragmented Self* is a great read.

One experience I had with The Sacred Trust was being taken through a process of spiritual dismemberment. This is not as worrying as it sounds. At any rate, I wasn't worried by it, and neither should you be. The idea is that you journey – it was to the Upper World this time – with the intention to ask for a dismemberment from a guide there who would appear to help you with the job.

Dismemberment is the idea that, safe in the Upper or Lower World, with your real body back at home, your spirit body can be taken apart and put back together again in a new and fresh way, as a kind of healing rebirth. The old is burnt away, and the new spirit body can emerge. No physical pain is involved; remember, this is all visualization, and it's seen as a loving act that spirit provides for you when you need it.

The way in which you are "dismembered" is entirely up to your guide. It's not pre-planned; you don't sit down beforehand and say, "I'd like to be cut up with scissors please!" You do the journey, you go to the guide and make the request, and the guide does the job. Your dismemberment might take the form of being turned to a pillar of sand and blown away in the breeze. It might be that you are dissolved in a lake. You might be exploded into space and become stardust. Or cut up with scissors, if you like. My experience was reasonably literal. I imagined/saw my spirit body being taken apart as if each part was joined to the rest of the body with poppers. Pop, pop, off came my knee, my shoulder and my arm, my head from my neck, etc. The pieces were like mannequin parts being piled up in the corner of the hut that all this was happening in. I didn't find this at all disturbing in my journey. It wasn't like there was blood or anything – although, sometimes, even though it's happening in the otherworld, you can feel certain sensations.

When it was all done, I was still me, regarding the pile of mannequin parts that my guide swept up unceremoniously (she is quite a no-nonsense guide) and added to her fireplace. It was an interesting insight also that I was still there as awareness without my spiritual body.

Then, it was time for my new body to arrive. Hurrah!

I watched as a perfect new body formed around "me", whatever I was at that point. It was like my old one but felt nicer, less stressy. The idea is that the new body will have none of your old knots or pains or obsessions and fixations; you can move forward now without anything holding you back.

The act of visualizing your body being destroyed in some way is, I suppose, quite weird and potentially scary. You might be thinking, *ugh, not for me!* That's fair. But, with these things it's all very much in the way you approach it and how the person guiding you through the technique in the real world holds the space to enable you to have your experience. Dismemberment is a very ancient spiritual technique belonging to shamans and is seen as a healing procedure. Unlike a Power Animal retrieval or a soul retrieval technique, a dismemberment allows a person to remake and optimize their whole spirit body.

This experience of spiritual dismemberment, of connecting to my Power Animals, and the soul retrieval sessions I undertook with Betsy the shamanic healer really helped me heal from the trauma of the early years of my son's life. They gave me strength, bravery and a place to go for healing whenever I needed it.

Because those early years were difficult. After a shaky start with his infection in hospital, I had become a highly anxious mother. Every time he picked up a normal bug, I was convinced it would land us back in hospital again – and in his first year, he must have had at least 10 colds or baby illnesses. It felt as though there was barely a week I wasn't dosing him up on Calpol.

When he was about three months old, he developed fairly severe eczema on his legs, arms and face. He'd just started to drop into a sleep routine that meant he'd wake up just twice a night and I felt like it was going well, but when the eczema started, it became six or seven wake-ups a night again. Sometimes he just wouldn't sleep at all; he was so agitated because of the itching. This went on for months and months with no improvement. My husband and I felt like we were banging our heads against a brick wall when it came to the doctors, who refused to prescribe my son any hydrocortisone because he was too little, and fobbed us off with moisturisers which did nothing at all.

I tried all the moisturisers. I tried the ones that mother and baby groups recommended. I tried the ones advertised on the internet: papaya extract, calendula, lavender. Oats in the bath. Oils in the bath. Cool baths. Bandaging. None of them worked. This eczema was hardcore. When I would breastfeed him, the sores on his face would start weeping. I was exhausted, he was exhausted, and every day was like walking over glass with a screaming baby and no sleep.

I felt like a thoroughly terrible mother for letting him go through all of this and not having any way of making it better; that was my job, and I was failing at it yet again. No one seemed to want to help us, and no one's kids had the same level of eczema as my son. For them it was easily solved with a little Sudocrem. In fact, the only kid that had it worse than my son was my cousin's little boy who, it turned out, was allergic to a lot of different foods, so when my cousin cut those food out of her diet (she was still breastfeeding) and removed the foods from his weaning menu, his skin improved. Yet, when I finally had my son tested for allergies, having asked and asked the doctor until they gave up and did it, none of the main ones – dairy, wheat, eggs – came back positive.[8]

Finally, I lost patience with conventional medicine that had utterly failed me on this issue and went to a local herbalist, who gave my son a course of tiny pills I had to dissolve in water. At this point, I would have tried feeding him a whole elephant if it had half a chance of working. He was almost a year old at this stage, and was still waking up through the night. I felt like my sanity was hanging in the balance.

Looking back, I'm amazed I was able to function at all. I know there were times when I was driving up and down the motorway near to us, waiting for my son to go to sleep in the back when there was no other way to get him to sleep, and my eyes would close for a moment or three as I sped along. Then, when he'd finally dropped off, I would drive back to my house

---

[8] Although much later I had him privately tested for food intolerances and he had wheat and cow's milk intolerances among others, so my intuition was right on that one.

and fall asleep myself, sitting up in the driver's seat for an hour, or sometimes two, mouth open and slumped, while he slept in the back. To this day, not one of my kind neighbours has ever mentioned the spectacle of my public sleeping to me, and that is why I love the British.

Anyway, about a week after starting with the herbalist, my son did a huge poo one night – so huge that I couldn't quite work out how it had come out of such a small child – and after that his skin seemed to improve a little. Around the same time, I managed to see a different doctor from the utterly useless ones I'd been seeing so far, who took one look at my son and said, "Yeah, moisturiser won't do anything for that. It's infected. I'll prescribe you some hydrocortisone."

One week after the huge poo and with the new cream, and the eczema was a thing of the past. Shortly after that, we successfully sleep trained our one-year-old and he started sleeping a lot better. Still not through the night – we didn't achieve that until he was four. But maybe two wake-ups a night, which we would have sold our souls for in that first year.

Gods. Be. Praised.

I don't know how many of you reading this have suffered the level of continued sleep deprivation that comes with being a new parent – probably many of you. It's a very hard thing to explain to anyone who hasn't been there because you can say the words to people, but words can in no way adequately represent the sheer brain-fogged, depressed, fearful, aching, bone-deep exhaustion that months and years of severely broken sleep bring. By "severely" I mean getting up around six times a night, every night, for a year or more.

The thing is with babies is that the night waking isn't just about getting up, serenely lying the baby back down in their cot and trotting back to your bed again. Oh no. Like many parents, I could expect to be up for around an hour or more every time, breastfeeding (he flatly refused to be bottle fed, so I couldn't share the feeding with my husband), nappy changing and then walking up and down the house patting his back or rocking him until he settled again (he also suffered terribly with wind, so would need to be walked or rocked for an hour after every feed. Every time. That's a lot of pacing up and down with an increasingly heavy, crying baby, if you consider that babies might feed 10 times in 24 hours during their early months or 4 to 8 times when they are bigger).

The other thing to say about having babies and young children is that even when you've got them through what I once heard someone call "the baby tunnel of hell" – for me, an excellent description – you aren't out of the woods. They still get ill all the time – especially if you send them to nursery – and then there's teething, separation anxiety and all the other weird stuff that kids do. And, importantly, all of these are things that keep them up at night too. Joy!

When my son was about three, he caught a mysterious virus that meant he wouldn't eat for about two to three months. No one was able to give us a diagnosis. It began with a high fever, a rash and vomiting and quickly developed into abdominal pain, listlessness and lack of appetite. Again, we were in and out of hospital as the doctors ummed and ahhed over whether this was appendicitis (it wasn't) or something else. Actually, we never found out what it was, but basically I kept my son alive on ice lollies and yoghurts and broke my own heart – again – in the process. He was so weak that he had to be carried to the toilet. Every day I hoped that day would be the one he ate and started to get stronger again; every day, he could do little more than lie on the sofa with me. It goes without saying that I am incredibly grateful to my boss at the time, who let me work from home a lot for those months.

Interestingly, this mystery illness occurred very soon after my son had started nursery a couple of mornings a week, which he hated. He'd been happily going to a lovely childminder a couple of days a week since he was one and I'd gone back to work part time (which saved my life, I'm sure. Not everyone likes going back to work after having a baby, but I LOVED it, and I will always be grateful to my amazing childminder who was just brilliant with my son and made it so easy for me). But he hated that nursery, big time. To be fair, it wasn't all that nice, but I was surprised: he'd been happy with his childminder and being away from me a couple of days a week for a while now. Why was this so much of a problem?

For whatever reason, it was, and when I dropped him off in the morning, he'd cling to me and cry. He refused to eat there. He wouldn't play. I felt awful, but other parents assured me that it was normal. He'd settle in a few weeks.

He didn't. Then, the mystery virus appeared and he was at home for a few months with me on the sofa. Now, I'm not saying for sure that his separation anxiety led to his virus, but there is a school of thought, as we've already touched on, that says that emotional trauma can cause physical symptoms. In this case, it's curious that the end result of this virus was that my son and I were almost literally joined at the hip for a few months as he recovered, the epitome of what a child with separation anxiety desires. This kid clearly gets his strong manifestation game from me.

During the long nights of sleeplessness and the long days worrying if my son would ever eat again (he did, thank God, and made a full recovery), I entertained some dark thoughts. I dreamed of running away and starting a new life somewhere else, on my own. I genuinely wondered whether I would ever have a normal night's sleep ever again. But most of all, I thought about those warmly lit depictions of breastfeeding mothers you see in films sometimes, where the mother is wearing some kind of flimsy nightdress, with full makeup and perfect long hair. You know, where the breastfeeding takes like five minutes and the baby doesn't scream its head off. Where you don't end up sleeping on the floor of the baby's room because if you leave the room, he will cry again.

I thought about all the crappy, smug books and articles I'd read about new motherhood, about taking time every day to do baby yoga or taking your baby out for babyccino or making organic food for the baby. I thought about all the mothers who had nice compliant babies they took on nice holidays or to baby groups because they didn't cry all the freaking time. I thought about all the terrible and conflicting advice I'd received: letting your baby sleep with you or not letting your baby sleep with you. Watching TV versus not watching TV. Spoon feeding versus baby-led weaning.

And I got more and more angry. In fact, I was furious.

Where was my cosy coffee morning? Where was my good little baby?

Fucking nowhere, that was where.

My kid, when he wasn't crying, itching and refusing to be bottle fed was, as an early walker, trashing the toddler music club by refusing to play along with the songs, running around the room and trying to pull apart the CD player and any other electronic device he could get his hands on. He was refusing to stay quiet in his pushchair in cafés and running straight toward the road in any kind of park. When we met other mums and toddlers for picnics, I spent 2 per cent of my time on the blanket with my friends and their delightfully stationary babies and 98 per cent of the time running after my son as he streaked through bushes and trees, down gravel paths and toward ponds and lakes. His favourite thing to do at home was repeatedly run up and down the length of the house pushing his wheeled suitcase, or run up and down the garden and eat the gravel. There was no gentle arts and crafts for me. And now, here he was again, seriously ill.

No one had told me about any of this. Think about any TV show where a character has a baby. Remember Rachel in *Friends*? How often do you even see Emma? She's always magically not there – at grandparents, or with a nanny. Rachel gets back to her life pretty quickly. I challenge you to think of any film or TV show that truly deals with the relentlessness, the exhaustion and the daily challenge of having babies and small children.

Obviously, I get that this is entertainment, and we all love *Friends* and its quippy wit and 90s nostalgia. Fine, fine. But what I'm saying is that the world around us does not prepare us for the reality of what having a baby actually is like, and I think that it should. And I think the reason that it doesn't is probably that a lot of people would not have babies if they knew. Perhaps controversially, I don't actually think this would be a terrible idea, as it goes. The planet is already massively overpopulated. And not everyone is cut out to be a parent. It's okay to say that.

I think there should be more support for new families. Some people employ doulas – holistic birth professionals – to help them with their baby's delivery and the early days at home after the birth, but that should be as standard for everyone. Everyone needs a live-in helper for at least a few months after having a baby, in my opinion. In an ideal world this would be a person who would cook, clean and look after the baby for a few hours here and there so you can sleep, or so you can go out without the baby for a while or do something truly radical like have a bath on your own. Most of all, it would be lovely to have someone there to assure you that you aren't going mad, to talk to, someone who can go with you to the doctor's surgery or the shops or (as kids get older) the mind-numbingly boring play parks and soft plays. Someone to just generally be around and say helpful things like "here's a cup of tea" and "I hung out the washing" or give you two minutes to brush your teeth.

Some of you might be thinking: 1. When is she going back to the shamanic journeying and 2. Didn't her husband do any of those things? Both of which are good questions. To answer 1: Very soon; stay with me, shamanism fans! To answer 2: Sure, when he was at home. But he was gone every weekday 8am to 6pm, and he even got home earlier than a lot of dads I knew who never saw their kids in the week at all. My own mother had passed away, and I was in a different city to my oldest friends, who were the ones I knew well enough to ask for help. I had few local friends and my work friends were all younger than me with no kids. I did see my dad weekly, which was a saving grace.

I was lonely, exhausted, depressed and constantly anxious about my son, who seemed super sensitive and open to everything that was going around, and I felt I was doing everything wrong.

Recently I was watching a Canadian TV series about four new mothers making the transition back to work, and coming to terms with their new lives. There's one episode where one of the characters comes across a bear in the forest while she's out with her baby in the pushchair. (It's Canada. Apparently bears in city forests are a thing there.) The bear growls threateningly at her, and instinctively she stands in front of the pushchair and screams as loud as she can back at the bear, even though she is, of course, terrified. You can see in her eyes in that moment a kind of primal rage and protectiveness. She roars back at the bear like a true animal herself: *Okay, you can come for him, but you'll have to go through me first.* It's a great scene.

The thing about motherhood is that it gives you this sense of primal strength and protectiveness over your children. I may not have faced a bear in my years as a mother, but I've gone to bat for my son many, many times. I've pushed for better support for him at school and with doctors; I've defended him from bullies and I've been on his side every single time he needed me, and I always will. Something kicks in when it comes to your children: the Mama Bear. It doesn't matter how chill you are as a person normally or how much you dislike confrontation. You will step up and do what is necessary to keep your children happy and healthy.

Was I doing everything wrong as a new mother? No! I was doing amazingly well, actually, but I didn't know that at the time. I was being Mama Bear, even though it was tough. I didn't feel tough at the time: I felt completely weak and vulnerable and heartbroken. But despite that, I fought for him, and I was there for him, and if I had to restrict myself to the sofa and miss work and weather that dark time with him then I would damn well do it.

Shamanic healing and journeying helped me process the trauma around my son's illnesses and my guilt at being a bad mother because it gave me an opportunity to reflect on those experiences. It also taught me how to draw strength from nature. I opened this chapter making fun of the "pretending to be animals" thing and, yes, it is very amusing. It's one of my chosen dinner party anecdotes. But, also, whatever reminds a struggling new mother of her bear-like strength and ability to protect her young can only be a good thing. For me, shamanic practices like power animal retrieval, where you journey to the Lower World to connect to a power animal essence you need at that point in your life, made me realize that I could tap into different modes or energies to help me. For me, it's empowering to know that I can be a Mama Bear and go to battle for my son if I need to. I don't want to have to be Mama Bear all the time – exhausting! And I have to remind myself that life is not all about dealing with moments of high stress. But it's good to know how to be a bear, and sometimes the time is right to stand protectively in front of our children and roar at whatever might hurt them.

Sometimes, too, if there's no one to do it for us, we have to be our own Mama Bear and protect ourselves from whatever wants to hurt us. Sometimes, it's good to dismember ourselves in a hut somewhere in the tundra and return from a shamanic journey refreshed and revived, feeling stronger and more purposeful. There is little help for new mothers, as I bemoaned earlier. Some might find comfort in a mother and baby café. Some might have helpful relatives or close friends that live nearby and who can move in and take the pressure off for a while.

I had none of that, but I did have that no-nonsense spirit woman, out in the desert, tending her horses, who was willing to make me tea whenever I would turn up at her door in a journey, needing her help. I had a partner who would take care of our son while I went away for weekends to meet up with strangers and learn all this weird stuff. And for those things I am thankful.

CHAPTER 8

A TRIAL BY BLOOD: BABALON, ENDOMETRIOSIS AND ME

What a chapter heading that is, eh? Sorry, guys.

So, like many women, I have always had a hate–hate relationship with my menstrual cycle. Ugh, I *hated* it. There was never a time it made me feel "womanly", whatever that means, unless "womanly" means "painful and angry" (which in fact it may do). I never got the hang of that whole "sacred mystery of the period" thing, despite having read the books claiming the mystical moon-based wonder of the menstrual cycle.

Fuck that shit.

I know that your menstrual cycle is there so that you can make babies. Yes, yes, I know. I know that. I had a baby! I made one. I saw it first-hand.

The wonder. The joy. The nausea. The compulsive eating of cream cakes. Quite honestly, I felt more like I had been invaded by an alien that had taken over my body. Don't even get me started on how, when you're pregnant, suddenly you become a host rather than a human in your own right. Everything is about the baby. All anyone cares about is that you're healthy because you're carrying the baby. Like you're a car that has to be kept in good condition because Burt Reynolds is about to thrash it within an inch of its life in *The Cannonball Run*.

On the plus side, at least you don't get your period for nine solid months (or maybe longer!) when you have a baby. And, you know, you make a whole person that you love. So there's that.

But, periods. What a waste of time. They really are literally the worst invention nature/God ever came up with. The patriarchy has made us ashamed of talking about them, of course, and don't get me wrong, I am firmly on the side of believing society should be much more accepting of women's bodies (in fact, let's have far more scientific research based on any bodies apart from white male ones – Caroline Criado Perez has written a great book about this[1]) and normalize what female bodies do. And what nonbinary and trans bodies do, come to that.

Yes, some of us bleed for at least a week every fucking MONTH, and whoever you are, that is a massive pain in the ass. Pain in the abdomen, actually, but whatever. You get used to it, you get on with your life, you don't go rollerblading in blinding white shorts (sorry, tampon advertisers) but you become friends with your hot water bottle and your ibuprofen and that's that for 35 to 40 years.

It's enough to make you utterly furious. And we are. Women. Furious, that is.

I was pretty furious all the time for many, many years, and it definitely wasn't helped by hormones, having to be incapacitated by my period, contraceptives that made me even more furious – and made it impossible to lose weight – everyday sexism (being told to "smile!" in the street. FUCK OFF AND DIE), the pay gap … you get it.

But one of the main reasons I was furious for quite a few years was that my body was betraying me.

---

[1] Caroline Criado Perez, *Invisible Women: Exposing Data Bias in a World Designed for Men*, Vintage

Legendary women's health campaigner Professor Mahmoud Fathalla, who, among many other honours and titles, worked for the UN and the World Health Organization advising on women's health, said in a report entitled 'Issues in Reproductive Health: Health and Being a Woman':

Being a woman has implications for health.[2]

He goes on to explain that people with a female reproductive system (as not everyone who suffers with gynaecological conditions identify as women) tend to suffer from different health concerns than those with a male reproductive system, and the most prevalent issues for those with a female reproductive system are ones concerning sexual and reproductive health. Basically, our reproductive system and all the issues related to it are our biggest problem. YAY.

When women, or those with a female reproductive system, suffer from the same issues as men, i.e. general disease, there is still a difference for women because of genetics, hormones or what he calls "gender-evolved lifestyle behaviour". (I take that to mean stuff women do or do not do as part of being women, i.e. more housework and caring for children, possibly less recreational drinking, certainly less walking around freely at night, or whatever). Last, he explains that women (and, I'd add, trans and nonbinary folks) are also far more subject to social health-related issues such as sexual abuse and domestic violence.

The professor reminds us:

The reproductive system, in function, dysfunction and disease, plays a central role in women's health. This is different from the case with men. A major burden of the disease in females is related to their reproductive function and reproductive system, and the way society treats or mistreats them because of their gender. While

---

2   www.un.org/womenwatch/daw/csw/issues.htm

more men die because of what one may call their "vices", women often suffer because of their nature-assigned physiological duty for the survival of the species, and the tasks related to it.

I'm sure that if Professor Fathalla was writing that report today (this was in 1997) he would also note that trans women suffer not only regular and continual threat from prejudice in society, but are also subject to a variety of other specific health concerns. *Being a woman has implications for health.*

My body was betraying me because I couldn't *stop* bleeding. Never mind one week a month; this was every day, no holidays, and it was *extreme* bleeding. Olympic-level bleeding. If vampires existed, I could have fed a family of four on an ongoing basis, no problem.

I know that sounds gross and, yes, I am trying to make a joke out of it but this was really, really not normal. I wasn't even having a period anymore because there was no end and no beginning. It was just always there, ruining my life in every single way you can imagine.

For instance, I often felt too weak and faint to get up (this level of blood loss frequently causes anaemia). I missed work because I was either too dizzy to commute, or I was bleeding so heavily that I literally could not get there without bleeding through any level of sanitary protection. And by "any level" I mean the toughest, thickest tampons and pads combined. I would go through a combined mega pad and tampon in an hour.

If I had been sitting down and then stood up, I would feel the blood gushing out of me. Those who have menstruated will know that a period can also involve womb lining and sometimes blood clots. I had blood clots falling out of me. I literally felt like I was dying. I remember being in the office at work one day, walking to the kitchen and feeling all the blood drain out of me. It was so bad I had to hang on to the shelves, make my way back to my desk and curl up underneath it. My boss sent me home.

As you can imagine, I had no sex life at this time, because not only was most of it not possible, I also didn't exactly feel very sexy. I was exhausted, in fact. It was not a fun time in my life, but unfortunately it lasted around two and a half to three years before I got it sorted – more on that later.

You may not know – I didn't before it happened to me – that thousands of people experience a range of conditions causing either excessive bleeding and intense, ongoing pain or hormonal mood conditions. We are starting to hear more about endometriosis now, but it's still early days and there are lots of other conditions like adenomyosis, PMDD (premenstrual dysphoric disorder), uterine fibroids and PCOS (polycystic ovary syndrome) that most people don't know about unless it happens to them. I've added some definitions here for those of you that may not be familiar. Knowledge is power and all that.

Endometriosis[3]

Endometriosis is when the kind of tissue that normally lines the uterus grows somewhere else. It can grow on the ovaries, behind the uterus, on the bowels, or on the bladder. Rarely, it grows in other parts of the body.

This "misplaced" tissue can cause pain, infertility and very heavy periods. The pain is usually in the abdomen, lower back or pelvic areas.

Here are some sobering stats from Endometriosis UK:[4]

- 1 in 10 women of reproductive age in the UK suffer from endometriosis.
- Around 10 per cent of women worldwide have endometriosis – that's 176 million worldwide. **176 MILLION.**
- The prevalence of endometriosis in women with infertility might be as high as 30–50 per cent.

---

[3] www.cdc.gov/reproductivehealth/womensrh/healthconcerns.html
[4] www.endometriosis-uk.org/endometriosis-facts-and-figures

- Endometriosis is the second most common gynaecological condition in the UK.
- Endometriosis affects 1.5 million women in the UK, which is similar to the number of women affected by diabetes.
- On average it takes eight years from onset of symptoms to get a diagnosis.
- Endometriosis costs the UK economy £8.2 billion a year in treatment, loss of work and healthcare costs.
- The cause of endometriosis is unknown and there is no definite cure.

Adenomyosis[5]

Adenomyosis is a condition where the lining of the womb grows into the muscle of the uterus.

No one knows why adenomyosis happens. It affects as many as one in ten women of reproductive age. It is more common in women aged 40–50 years and who have had children.

The most common symptoms are:

- Heavy, painful or irregular periods
- Pre-menstrual pelvic pain and feelings of heaviness/ discomfort in the pelvis

Less common symptoms are:

- Pain during sexual intercourse
- Pain related to bowel movements

About one third of women experience few or no symptoms; other women suffer with many effects. It can also affect other aspects of a woman's life including her general physical health and emotional wellbeing. Symptoms will stop after the menopause.

---

[5] www.nbt.nhs.uk/our-services/a-z-services/gynaecology/adenomyosis

Adenomyosis does not appear to decrease the chance of pregnancy; however, it is linked to an increased risk of miscarriage and premature birth.

PMDD[6]

Premenstrual dysphoric disorder (PMDD) is a very severe form of premenstrual syndrome (PMS). It causes a range of emotional and physical symptoms every month during the week or two before a menstrual cycle. It is sometimes referred to as "severe PMS".

There are so many symptoms for this one that the website I visited, MIND (a prominent UK-based mental health charity), had to split them into two categories: physical and emotional.

Physical and behavioural experiences are:

- Breast tenderness or swelling
- Pain in your muscles and joints
- Headaches
- Feeling bloated
- Changes in your appetite, such as overeating or having specific food cravings
- Sleep problems

Emotional experiences are:

- Mood swings
- Increased anger or conflict with people around you
- Feeling upset or tearful
- Lack of energy
- Less interest in activities you normally enjoy
- Feeling hopeless
- Suicidal feelings
- Feeling angry or irritable

---

6   www.mind.org.uk/information-support/types-of-mental-health-problems/premenstrual-dysphoric-disorder-pmdd/about-pmdd/

- Feeling anxious
- Feeling tense or on edge
- Feeling overwhelmed or out of control
- Difficulty concentrating

PCOS[7]

PCOS stands for Polycystic Ovary Syndrome. This happens when a woman's ovaries or adrenal glands produce more male hormones than normal. One result is that cysts develop on the ovaries. Women with PCOS are at increased risk of developing diabetes and heart disease. Symptoms may include:

- Infertility
- Pelvic pain
- Excess hair growth on the face, chest, stomach, thumbs or toes
- Baldness or thinning hair
- Acne, oily skin or dandruff
- Patches of thickened or darkened skin

Uterine fibroids[8]

Uterine fibroids are the most common non-cancerous tumours in women of childbearing age. Fibroids are made of muscle cells and other tissues that grow in and around the wall of the uterus, or womb. The cause of fibroids is unknown. Symptoms of fibroids include:

- Heavy or painful periods or bleeding between periods
- Feeling "full" in the lower abdomen
- Urinating often
- Pain during sex
- Lower back pain
- Reproductive problems, such as infertility, multiple miscarriages, or early labour

---

[7]   www.cdc.gov/reproductivehealth/womensrh/healthconcerns.html
[8]   www.cdc.gov/reproductivehealth/womensrh/healthconcerns.html

As we learn about the symptoms and facts around these conditions, you'll notice a few recurring themes. One is that they are very common – endometriosis and adenomyosis, for example, affect roughly one in ten women, and that's not even factoring in fibroids, PCOS, PMDD and the other conditions I haven't even listed here. Have you also noticed that a common feature of many of these conditions is pain, bleeding and generally horrendous symptoms? I have!

The third common theme is that the medical community apparently know jack shit about gynaecological health, which most women who have gone to their GP with excessive pain and bleeding in the past thousand years will confirm.[9]

I joined an adenomyosis support group on Facebook. In that group alone – there are lots of others – there are, at the time of writing, 12,000 members.

Look at the facts listed here. There is no known cure for endometriosis or adenomyosis, apart from the menopause (yay! The menopause! Don't even get me started on that). The cause of fibroids is unknown. The cause of adenomyosis and endometriosis is unknown. Why do some women experience PMDD, or other conditions such as postnatal depression? What causes PCOS? What cures it?

NO ONE KNOWS.

How do these two facts coexist? How is it possible that perhaps half of all women ON THE PLANET (maybe more!) will experience at least one gynaecological condition in their lives that will seriously affect their mental health and quality of life – which will likely inflict excessive pain, discomfort and inconvenience and can in many cases cause significant problems with fertility?

---

[9]   Look, I respect the hell out of the medical community; I appreciate our free healthcare and I am grateful for it. But the fact remains that there is a gulf of research and understanding that needs to be filled when it comes to women's health.

How is it possible that the medical community don't have any good answers for women suffering with conditions that are this prolific?

Yes, this made me furious (as furious as I could feel with no energy, anyway). It still makes me furious. I am angry about this.

Let me tell you what I was offered for my debilitating condition.

First attempt: I was told I had "heavy periods", the standard doctor's answer to basically any gynaecological query, it seems. I tried to explain that I thought something was seriously wrong. The doctor wearily prescribed me the contraceptive pill. I hadn't been on the pill since my late twenties and I'd really enjoyed not being fat and depressed in the intervening years, so I wasn't happy to be back on it, but I took it. The doctor did not mention any of the conditions described above.

It lessened the bleeding to the level of a normal period for a couple of months, and then stopped working completely and I was back to square one.

Second attempt: I paid to see a private GP. He was much more sympathetic, which kind of comes with the price tag. He gave me a different pill, a hardcore progesterone one, that was strong enough to stop the bleeding. I was only allowed to take it for a week and then we'd see if the bleeding returned. I could have told him that it would, but he seemed to believe that might do it. He also gave me a scan that confirmed I had PCOS. He suggested it might be possible I had adenomyosis and explained what that was.

After a week blissfully blood-free on the progesterone, but also a week of crying on and off like a mournful tap, the bleeding returned. I called the private GP again and he prescribed me a different, lower dose progesterone medication.[10] It didn't work in the slightest.

I returned and saw a different private GP who prescribed me a different, "body identical" progesterone that is also used as

---

[10] For reference, this was Cerelle.

an HRT treatment. "Body identical" means that the hormones contained in it are derived in nature[11] and are identical to the hormones in the body. Synthetic hormones means that they are created in laboratories, not derived from nature. She explained that synthetic and body-identical progesterone affect people very differently, and the body identical one she was now prescribing me would be much better for my mood. She jokingly acknowledged that norethisterone, the extra-strong progesterone I had previously been prescribed, was notorious for making women suicidal. Hahaha, all the LOLs. Suicide. Hilarious.

Let's not linger on the question of why *any* drugs exist which have SUICIDE among their side effects. Let's just keep prescribing them to women with no other option, eh? *Great.*

You can tell in this chapter that I am as mad as hell, and I really am. I'm angry about all this, both from my own perspective but more for all the millions of women out there that are still suffering. I'm sorry that I'm less amusing (if I was ever amusing) than in other parts of the book. I am leading up to something here so bear with me, but also let's acknowledge that RAGE is a natural reaction to things being crappy.

Rage is part of our healing process. It's important to feel our feelings, especially when they are the socially less approved feelings like sorrow, rage, jealousy and desire. Rage is a special no-no for women. Sometimes I think what I'd like to do is hold some RAGE DAYS especially for women – and anyone identifying as a woman – where we can all get together in a remote location, or maybe in a soundproofed soft-play room (safe to pound on the walls with your fists) and scream our brains out in a safe environment. Afterwards we'd have a nice meal and a good sleep. There could be medical specialists and therapists on hand.

It's also important to note that, on our healing journey, whatever form that takes, whether it involves alternative therapies or not, we deserve to *actually get the healing we need*

---

[11] In the case of HRT, often from yams, I believe. Let's all eat yams and be happy.

from the medical profession. Medicine and surgery can and should be part of our healing journey when appropriate. Again, I'm going to say that many times, people get what they need and that's great. But, often, not when a faulty uterus is concerned. Certainly not in my experience, anyway.

So, this slightly more helpful GP prescribed me this body-identical progesterone called Utrogestan which she thought would help. She also suggested I ask my GP to refer me to a gynaecologist to look into the problem further and told me that the only real cure for this problem was a hysterectomy. Instinctively, I didn't want that, but at the same time I was already pretty sick and tired of the bleeding.

Please note that so far this process had taken months.

Utrogestan got off to a shaky start with some intense period pain and very heavy bleeding in the first week, but then it started to actually work. The bleeding stopped for about three weeks out of four. Gods be praised! It also didn't make me suicidal OR particularly depressed – a win – AND you have to take it before you go to bed because it knocks you out. So I got great sleep too.

I took Utrogestan for a few months, but then slowly the bleeding started to come back. It wasn't much, just a little every day, but it was still constant and enough to be annoying and continue to restrict my sex life. On the plus side, I wasn't in danger of anaemia anymore and could go to the office without major preparations, tampon- and pad-wise.

I stuck it out with the Utrogestan. It was still better than the previous pills, and life was better than it had been for a long time, so I did what many of us do, and accepted a less than perfect situation as the best possible. Better the devil you know.

I got on with life, but the thing with this drug was that it could suddenly stop working here and there with no warning. Fun times!

For example, once I was with my son in the car on our way to a children's literary festival at which I was supposed to be looking after an author. I'd brought my son along to make a day of it.

Unfortunately, as we sat at traffic lights just outside of Barnes in leafy southwest London, I felt a sudden warm flood of blood soak my jeans. Frantically stuffing tissues into my knickers while sitting at traffic lights was not my finest moment, and neither was drying out my underwear and the crotch of my jeans in a literary festival green room toilet.

Another time, I was working away for a few days with another author doing a school tour. While we waited for our train home at Sheffield railway station, another sudden flood of blood rushed out of me, soaking my jeans (another pair ruined). I had to run to the toilets, clean up what I could, accept an emergency tampon from the slightly freaked-out author in question and endure several hours on the train home, hoping it wouldn't happen again and that I wouldn't soak the train seat.

I went back to the GP again and asked to be referred to a gynaecologist. She refused, instead giving me the choice between what's called ablation and a hormonal IUD (inter uterine device) called the Mirena coil. I asked again. *I really think I'd like a hysterectomy. I don't want any more children and I just can't cope with the bleeding anymore.*

I didn't want to mess around with more "possible" solutions. By now, I knew the only complete solution to my problem was a hysterectomy. At first, I'd hated the idea. I'd felt it would make me less of a woman. And I had a guilty feeling that I shouldn't have a hysterectomy because it would be kind of anti-goddess. Like I'd be less connected to the goddess energies of life-giving in some deeply primal way. No, I'd never really related to the idea that having periods made me somehow connected to the divine, but the concept can be very persuasive. In my opinion, having a uterus has absolutely no relationship to your relationship with goddess energy. In fact, if I was feeling especially cynical, I'd say that telling women that their debilitating gynaecology brings them closer to God is manipulative, disempowering bullshit aimed at getting women to accept their lot without complaining. Ask girls who can't access education because of period poverty how empowering it is and I think you'd get the answer "not very".

Neither of those things were true, as it turns out, but that was genuinely how I felt at the time, and I don't think it's uncommon to fear a loss of "womanliness" – whatever that is – when thinking about a hysterectomy.

The GP refused. She explained that they'd refer me to a gynaecologist to talk about possibly having a hysterectomy after I'd tried either the ablation or the Mirena coil.

Time stretched out before me in a bloody mess – months and months more of waiting, hanging around, bleeding, while the NHS tried yet another halfway measure. I said I'd think about it (I knew I didn't want either) and went away to do some research, as I'd heard bad things about both – all the time relying on my often-faulty hormone medication which had more and more frequent blips.

In my Facebook group for adenomyosis sufferers, I asked about people's experience of the Mirena coil and ablation. You may be wondering what ablation is at this point, so let me enlighten you.

Ablation is where a doctor sticks a laser up your vagina and burns off the internal layers of your uterus while you're awake.

Yes, you heard me right. Another medieval treatment for women's bodies from the scientific community.

So, not only are they okay with prescribing us hormones that make us suicidally depressed – AND HAVEN'T FOUND ANYTHING BETTER DESPITE IT BEING 2022 – they're also fine with LITERALLY BURNING OUT OUR WOMBS.

Fuck. No.

No way was anyone burning my endometrial wall off, thank you very much. A friend of mine had it done for fibroids and she said while they did it there was a smell of burning meat in the room. Again, I'm compelled to wonder whether there's a comparable medical procedure for men, and I just can't think of one. Yet another indignity women are expected to put up with, along with the menstrual cycle, childbirth and the menopause.

In my Facebook group, several women had taken the ablation option to stop their heavy bleeding and pain, but no one had anything good to say about it. In many cases the bleeding had got worse rather than better.

I decided against the ablation. I also didn't like the sound of the Mirena coil (like a normal coil, an implanted device that makes your body believe it's pregnant and hence theoretically stops you having a period or conceiving), which had worked okay for some women, but again, the majority of experience was bad. Again, the Mirena coil had made bleeding heavier, had created additional infections, had sometimes got stuck inside the uterus, and had made the pain worse.

I was still considering the options a few months later when Utrogestan stopped working altogether.

Picture the scene: It was a sunny June day, it was my son's birthday and we were out with his best friend and her mum, Katie. The kids were having a cycle ride in a forest and Katie and I were walking and having a catch-up. Covid had been with us a few months and an outside play date with one friend was pretty much the best birthday option the kid had.

Please also note that this was a forest, not a park, so there were no public toilets. Just trees.

As the kids cycled off into the distance and Katie and I walked along a forest path, I felt the familiar gush announce itself.

Fuck, not *again*.

Fortunately, I had my handbag with me. I had to run into the forest, leaving Katie to keep an eye on the kids, undo my jeans and stuff two super-strength tampons into my vagina as fast and accurately as possible and then get dressed again before any dog walkers came by.

Dog walkers *did* come by. Unbelievable! Like, suddenly all of Surrey is out and about in the forest? Why weren't they at home? It was a lockdown, for god's sake! Being a middle-aged woman worked for me on this occasion. I guess the dog walkers didn't suspect me of being a pervert, and walked on.

It wasn't one of my greatest moments, if I'm honest. I had to pretend to be looking in fascination at the tree I was standing partly behind and hope that they didn't notice my jeans weren't done up.

Also, by the way, wearing two large tampons at a time is hugely uncomfortable and I don't recommend it, but it was an emergency and I didn't want to ruin my son's birthday by not letting him have his play date.

I was disappointed Utrogestan had stopped working. I'd really enjoyed that lovely medicated sleep every night.

I rang the GP from the forest in tears, feeling completely at the end of my tether. Luckily, I spoke to a different doctor from the evil one who had refused to refer me to a gynaecologist. This GP arranged a prescription for the dreaded suicidal-feelings-inducing norethisterone again, but, this time, I had to take two every day. At that stage, I didn't have a choice anymore.

I asked this different GP to take pity on me and refer me to a gynaecologist, which she agreed to do. Finally, someone was listening to me – it had only taken about five tries.

Let's sidestep the detailed gynaecological minutae of my life for a moment here and talk a little about the "Babalon" part of the title of this chapter.

While all this was going on, I had started writing a novel. In fact, I'd started writing it just before the crazy excessive bleeding began.

It wasn't my first novel. I'd written quite a few already and had them published to various levels of success. But, as I wrote this one, enraged by my experiences of generally being a woman in the world, now furious with my body which felt like it was trying to kill me, and desperately sad about the state of the world in which women were consistently abused, unheard and denied control over their bodies, I started to intuitively connect to a "dark" goddess, Babalon, who so far I knew little about.

What is the dark feminine, I hear you ask? Like The Morrigan, who for me provided a place of support among other women and an acknowledgement of my pain and anger, Babalon is an energy, described as a goddess by some, that represents the totality of existence and non-existence. Many of the books about Babalon I had read at this point and the conversations I had about her put her in this "dark feminine" category. In our patriarchal society, we have lived in a binary mode of light = good, dark = bad for thousands of years. In our binary world, values are assigned on both sides: light/male/positive/healing/sun/good versus dark/female/negative/mystery/blood/pain/moon/bad. We can see this in the way that the image of the witch has been considered evil in our society, and in the story of Adam and Eve, with Eve causing the downfall of humanity because of her fascination with the mysterious serpent (and, by the way, receiving the punishment for all women for eternity: in the Bible God says, "I will greatly multiply your pain in childbearing; in pain you shall bring forth children, yet your desire shall be for your husband, and he shall rule over you.")

Yeah, it was all our own fault. All that blood and pain and domestic abuse.

eyeroll

The dark feminine is also the goddess Persephone who travels to the underworld to become its queen. The dark feminine is the darkness, the pain, the mystery and the magic of being alive that there is no solution to, other than sitting with it. The dark feminine is acknowledging that death is a natural – and essential – part of life. Life cannot always be light. Life cannot always expand and progress. There has to be decay. There has to be an end. There are times of restriction, reflection, stillness, inertia. You cannot will everything to happen in the way you want it to. The universe is bigger than you.

In fact, I don't know how I first came across Babalon. All I really remember is that I started having some pretty dark dreams at this time, about snakes and halls of reptiles I was terrified of but which I knew I had to travel through to get to the other side.

Snakes are one of the oldest symbols of health, power and mysticism, and relate to our deep past as humans, perhaps both from an evolutionary point of view from when we were all reptiles, or from those early days when the human mind became programmed to fear predators such as snakes. Snakes appear as power symbols in all manner of ancient cultures, such as in the caduceus of Hermes in Greek mythology, representing magic, and the rod of Asclepius the healer, also a Greek god (the single snake curling around the tree branch), which is our symbol for medicine now.

In the Old Testament[12] God punished the Israelites for complaining as they wandered in the desert by visiting them with a plague of poisonous snakes. As a cure, he told Moses to make a bronze snake and wrap it around his staff: anyone who looked at the snake would be cured. There's also the famous serpent in the Garden of Eden, of course, who guards the arcane knowledge of the Tree of Life, and the snake of *kundalini*, the erotic feminine *Shakti* power we can harness in our bodies and energy fields. I also always look at the caduceus of Hermes and immediately think of DNA: the double helix symbol, the twin snakes twisting around and around each other, much like the way one is taught to envisage the snake-like coil of energy that represents kundalini energy rising and twisting up the central pillar of the body.

Snakes aren't obviously associated with Babalon – typically she is depicted as the luxuriously dressed Whore of Babylon in the biblical imagery, riding a many-headed beast, or as a goddess-like figure in the Strength card in the tarot (also named Lust) where she holds the jaws of a lion closed, or rests a restraining hand on the animal in some way. But snakes are also NOT associated with Her either. For instance, the ancient tantric practices of the priests and priestesses of the *Vama Marg* and other related schools of mystical union with the gods, are centred on the snake-like kundalini practices, and in Thelema, Babalon's sex/death energy of empowerment has a distinctly tantric element to it.

The goddess Babalon was originally "discovered" by Dr John Dee, Queen Elizabeth I's magician, in his magical experiments in the 16th century. Later, she was integrated into Aleister

---

12   Numbers 21: 4-9

Crowley's system of magic, Thelema, in the early 20th century. Crowley identified her with the Whore of Babylon in the Book of Revelation of the Bible.

She is also linked to the goddess Inanna, an ancient Mesopotamian goddess associated with love, beauty, sex, war, justice and political power. Inanna was later worshipped by the Akkadians, Babylonians and Assyrians under the name Ishtar; both are prototypes for the kind of goddess Babalon has become in the world at large at this point in time: that of sexual and gender liberation, freedom and the power of the dark feminine. Other goddesses such as Lilith (who is often associated with snakes) are sometimes aligned with Babalon and others by those interested in deities that lend themselves to an anti-patriarchal modus operandi.

Lilith tends to be thought of as a feminist force or symbol nowadays because in the Bible, where she comes from, she was Adam's wife before Eve but was cast out of Eden, becoming a baby-killing demon because she "refused to lie under Adam". Her "baby-killing" status (and lack of inclination to be sexually submissive to her male partner) is often read these days by feminists as representing her identity as a female who exercises reproductive control.[13]

Aleister Crowley described Babalon as the holiest of holies who was simultaneously the magical whore goddess and the goddess of the stars and creator of the universe. Crowley also saw Babalon as a catalyst for women's changing role in society. Characterizing her human representatives as Scarlet Women, freely liberated sexual women, he believed that this was a role that real-life women could – and should – embody.

Bearing in mind that he was writing at the turn of the 20th century, you could say that Crowley foresaw the sexual revolution of the 1960s, and the rise of feminism, by many decades. Though he himself remains a controversial figure, it seems important

---

[13] wiccanrede.org/2016/04/the-coming-forth-of-babalon/ is a useful overview for that point of view.

that his message regarding the role of the Scarlet Women was that women – and indeed all humans – should be free to express themselves sexually. "Should" is a very idealistic word, though. In a world where 50 per cent of the population's health needs are under-served by research, medication and capacity, there is a much higher barrier to sexual freedom for women, trans and nonbinary folks than there is for men. Further, there are obvious repercussions for sexual freedom in countries where being gay is still against the law.

Yes, we *should* all be free to express our sexuality, but cultural, social and structural inequalities still stand in our way.

Crowley's reason for espousing this view must have been the knowledge that unless a person is connected to their sexual power and is able to use and control their physical energy and energy field proficiently, then they will have difficulty reaching the enlightenment of connection to a higher power. For him, this was the universal energy of Nuit, who is represented as the void of space and beyond: complete nothingness. In Thelema, Crowley's philosophical-magical system, the main goal of an adherent is to achieve knowledge of and conversation with one's own Holy Guardian Angel via a long process of spiritual purification – which, one could say, fits in rather well with the general concept of healing. When one manages to talk to one's Holy Guardian Angel, one is told one's life purpose and any secrets or insights that the Angel might want to confer.

Babalon could be said to represent the acceptance of all things. Because of her association with Crowley's Scarlet Woman, she stands for sexual liberation, and more and more she is being adopted by trans and nonbinary groups too as a goddess for all. One of her names is the Holy Whore because she loves everything the universe has to offer: all the beauty, and all the horror. She is rage, and she is radical acceptance. She loves all bodies and for Babalon, like it says in the Charge of the Goddess, a poetic call to the goddess within traditional Wicca, *all acts of love and pleasure are my rituals.* Within Babalon we find a radical acceptance of the totality of everything: all the awfulness of humanity, all the good. All the universe and all the void. Everything of everything.

So that's Babalon, in a pretty large nutshell.

After a series of some mega synchronicities in my life at that time where I kept seeing people I knew online talk about the goddess Babalon and kept seeing books about Babalon in shops, I got the message and started to investigate Her. I found that some people had adopted Her as a kind of rage-filled protectress of women's bodies, and I related hard to that. My body was much in need of protecting, both from itself and from the medical community that wanted to burn bits of it off. Never mind the fact that those same people also didn't seem to have any answers for why it was malfunctioning to such an alarming degree.

In writing my novel, I felt the energy of Babalon: rage and rage on behalf of other women and vulnerable people who may have been persecuted. I wrote about it. I felt it. My illness continued throughout: continual bleeding, fatigue, anaemia. I sat with it, experiencing the initiations of the dark goddess, which is acceptance of death and endings and the underworld. I connected with others who had also connected with Babalon, including my friend Lou Hotchkiss-Knives, who, rather wonderfully, fronts a riot grrrl-style punk band wholly dedicated to Babalon called Husbands n' Knives.[14] This inspired part of my novel, which is told by three women, all experiencing that Babalon energy in different ways. One of them is in a riot grrrl-style band – it was too good not to put in, and anyway, that style of music perfectly captures the energy we were feeling at the time: rebellious, feminist, confrontational. For all the characters in the book, the experience of Babalon is transformational – as it has been in my life, too.

I had more dreams about having to navigate a horrifying museum of reptilian monsters. Again and again I walked through that dream museum, feeling the fear bubble up inside me. The

---

[14] If you like Hole and Bikini Kill, you're going to love them.

monsters were behind glass, but I was still terrified of them. Just the sight of them, the size of them, dinosaur-like, filled me with a sense of doom. I continued writing my book, which was turning out to be a story of blood and sex and revenge, of magic and women's liberation, and of the failures of power.

I let myself go into the dark. I tried hard to accept what my body was doing. I collected up everything life was demonstrating to me about suffering – and everything else I had experienced – and sat with it. Tried not to judge it, or analyse it.

I realized that, with the bleeding, I had to accept that no one knows why many gynaecological conditions occur.

Did that make me angry? Yes.

Does it still make me angry? Yes.

Is it okay to be angry? Yes, and it's good to express that anger.

Can I, in some small way, use my knowledge and anger and experience to do something for someone else? Yes. I'm doing it now.

Did I have to accept that this was happening to me, look it in the face and still try to love the fact that it was part of my life? Because I am alive, and this is part of life? Yes.

Babalon is the simultaneous radical acceptance of the fact that no one knows why many gynaecological conditions occur, and the rage that no one knows why many gynaecological conditions occur. Babalon is the simultaneous radical acceptance of the fact that I had to watch my mother die in agonising pain and confusion, and the rage that I had to watch my mother die in agonising pain and confusion. Babalon is the simultaneous radical acceptance of fearing that your newborn baby will die, and the determined rage that makes you do whatever is necessary to keep him alive.

Babalon is the terrible, radical acceptance of all the abuse women, children and vulnerable people receive in this hell hole of a world we live in, and the determined rage of every person that seeks to protect them from it.

One day, I dreamed that reptile museum had turned into a children's water park, and I sailed down a water slide, away from the caged beasts. Maybe that meant that I had accepted what was happening to me. Maybe that meant I had accepted Babalon. Maybe it meant I had accepted myself. I don't entirely know. But I wrote that novel, and finished it. Later, I found a small publisher that published it. And that was something.

CHAPTER 9

SCREAMING ON AN INDUSTRIAL ESTATE WITH STRANGERS: BREATHWORK

Six breaths is all it takes to move on.

This is what Matthew and Adam, two ex-builders, now breathwork facilitators, explained to us as we sipped tea in a room above a mechanic's workshop on an industrial estate.[1]

In terms of glamorous locations, I really felt like I'd hit the big time. When driving in, I'd parked in the forecourt of a paint manufacturer, and when looking for the place I'd been told to find, walked past several men in overalls smoking cigarettes. The industrial estate in question backed onto a canal which was pretty in parts but – as in this part – grimy and covered in graffiti in others.

To get to the breathwork workshop I had to go through a mechanic's workshop, with the mechanic (Matthew's dad) doing his accounts at a desk covered in spanners.

Above, there was a room with a comfy sofa, amethyst and citrine towers and framed pictures of Sai Baba. Incense was

---

[1] For those of you playing Healing Location Bingo through this book, HOUSE!

burning. I almost did a double take. I was offered a cup of tea and a custard cream. This was more familiar ground than the industrial estate outside.

I'd paid (a nominal amount) to be here for a three-hour workshop session, and I was curious to learn more about breathwork. There were only three of us taking the workshop, and two instructors.

Now, generally speaking, I don't run into people that I find truly difficult very often, because my work and lifestyle usually finds me among people I like, or with at least some common ground between us. In fact, I probably don't agree with many people about the minutae of their views and ethics, but I wouldn't let that come between us. You can't expect people to be completely the same as you, and unless that person has actual, real responsibility for a situation you passionately feel should be changed (can they solve world hunger? Can they close Guantanamo Bay detention camp? Do they have a presentation slot at the next world climate conference that would benefit from your insight? Are they on the local council?) then you can disagree with them but you still have to accept that they will have opinions that you find stupid. At the same time, you can go ahead and make the world better in the way you think it should be.

I am a great believer in the phrase "opinions are like bums: everyone has one". Further, life is much easier when you don't have to experience the nasty ones en masse.

That's not to say that everyone with a beautiful bottom deserves to have their opinion promoted above others, of course. Henry Cavill's arse is beautiful enough to merit its own plinth in Trafalgar Square, but I'm not saying he should necessarily be consulted on matters of public safety or solutions to colony collapse disorder.[2]

What I'm saying is, I am usually able to perceive that someone's opinion on a subject has little relationship to the reality of the

---

[2] Although, if he was willing, I'm sure he'd have something good to say. Ah, Henry.

situation, which is defined by facts and changed by action, not opinions. Opinions can sometimes (but definitely not always) be changed by information, whether that information is "fake news" or propaganda, academic research or reading a book. But sometimes, my gods, someone pushes my buttons and no amount of rationalization is going to help.

One of the other people in the workshop was an ex-military man whose name I've actually forgotten, so let's call him Carl. Carl was one of those middle-aged white men who have apparently decided that everyone in the room is interested in what he has to say.

One of the unintended effects of telling the room your life story in a loud voice is that you never know when someone will be recounting your badly thought-out opinions (which are, nonetheless, yours and you have a right to them) in a book to demonstrate how frigging irritating, entitled and sexist some men can be.

Sorry, Carl.

In fact, Carl was an interesting guy, because he had served in the army for many years and now ran a therapy programme for ex-soldiers with PTSD. He'd come along to the breathwork session with a view to maybe doing breathwork with his group. Breathwork is actually perfect for PTSD and trauma gained from combat and conflict situations: it can deal with that big stuff, and provide a safe arena for people to express difficult emotions and memories. So, Carl was actually doing brilliant things and I was really interested in what he had to say about the mental health of ex-soldiers. It was just that he was also, in my opinion, a massive dick.

Why did I feel that about him, so viscerally? Part of it was definitely because of his racist views, which apparently he felt at ease throwing around the room. Part of it was also because he described his wife's reiki practice as "sparkly fairy stuff", repeatedly described himself as "roughty-tuffty" and described all the rough-and-tough soldier things he was trained to do (it wasn't "kill a man with a pencil" but it was in that ballpark) and told us about how he was preparing his sons for the apocalypse by teaching them to hunt and kill animals. He was pushing a number of my buttons, certainly with his loud-mouth manner, which I always hate. But then I took a step back and thought, *Okay. What is this? What is this, really?*

I don't know about you, but I take the view that on the rare occasion I do happen to meet someone whose views I find utterly repellent, I try to see it as a gift from God/the universe. Like, this meeting is an opportunity for me to release my opposition and anger, the feelings that this person evokes, and if being in someone's presence literally makes me beside myself with fury, then there has to be something more going on inside me – it's not just about this person.

Ordinarily I operate in a very female-dominated environment. I work in a female-dominated industry and I socialize with people with the same generally liberal mindset to me. What the universe seemed to be giving me was a three-hour window of enforced proximity within controlled conditions with The Toxic Masculine. I decided to see it as an opportunity. And I ran with it.

I'd heard about breathwork for a long time, in fact, as it was another therapy taught by the group I'd done my original reiki level one and two with. Yet, until now, I hadn't been compelled to try it. I don't know if it was a psychic impulse that something bad was coming and I wouldn't have an opportunity again to do healing in person for a while (this was the month before the Covid lockdown started), but something attracted me to the mention of the low-cost workshop in an email. I signed up.

Breathwork is a fast-breathing method that puts you in a kind of trance state where it is easier to express emotions. The concept is that breath regulates our perceptions and emotions, and when it's sped up to a certain rhythm for limited periods of time, it makes it easier for your unconscious to release stored trauma. Matthew and Adam had both turned their lives around with breathwork (you can read my interview with Matthew about his life-changing experience of breathwork after this chapter) and explained to us how trauma is stored in the unconscious, building up over time so that our systems have to commit more and more energy to dealing with it and maintaining it on an unconscious level.

Matthew gave us the image of the huge warehouse that the Ark of the Covenant gets lost inside in *Raiders of the Lost Ark*. Remember that scene? It's at the end of the film, Indiana Jones has fought the Nazis who want the power of the Ark for their nefarious purposes, and the US government official assures Indy that the Ark is being analysed by its "top guys" as they speak. Then we see the Ark being packed into a wooden crate labelled TOP SECRET ARMY INTEL DO NOT OPEN and wheeled into a warehouse full of identical crates. The camera pans out and we see that the warehouse goes on forever. It's utterly vast, and we know that Indy was right: the US government aren't going to do anything with the Ark but sit on it, just like (presumably) they've sat on the millions of other priceless treasures and/or supernatural weird shit and phenomena in the rest of those crates, squirrelled away from the public eye.

Say what you like about *Raiders of the Lost Ark*'s dated cultural references, but this scene is a brilliant representation of the unconscious and all the trauma and old patterning stored in there (and any movie that dresses Harrison Ford in a natty 1930s suit and hat at the end has my vote).

Imagine, for a moment, your own unconscious, full of boxes. Wouldn't it be a relief to let go of some of them? All those old thoughts, fears, patterns you didn't even know were in there? Imagine how much more room you'd have for new things – fresher ways of being, healthier patterns – more aligned to your wellbeing. Or just the emotional space to *be*.

Okay. I was ready for this. To be honest, even though I loved this metaphor about the warehouse and the Ark of the Covenant, I didn't really expect anything to happen to me during the breathing except the state of pure bliss Adam had described. Sometimes, if there's nothing to dump out of the warehouse, you get to a blissful state of just being, he'd said. Being with the universe. Seeing the workings of the universe in their divine glory. Knowing that you are a divine, beautiful part of creation.

Yeah, I was up for that. I'd been a reiki practitioner for years now. I'd been a practising witch. I had Done Stuff. I gazed at my fellow workshop-takers with a kind of sickening humanitarian humility. They might have some stuff come up. I knew that I wouldn't because I'd already cried in community centres so many times now. I'd bawled on treatment tables. I had given myself up to healing so many times. If I wasn't whole by now, then I was close.

Oh, kind reader, I feel like you know where this is going.

I laid down on a yoga mat, my head on a pillow, and arranged a blanket over me. So far, so cosy. Matthew turned on some music: a specially curated playlist. Some classical music began. I started the breathing, following the pattern Adam was demonstrating. It was a little hard to get used to, but then I kind of got the hang of it. It was like forcing yourself to be out of breath.

We listened to emotive music – Bach to Eminem – and did the breathing.

Within a few minutes, I started to feel an emotion bubble up inside me. I kept breathing.

Apparently, there is a difference between the breathing method we were doing and what's called holotropic breathwork, which is designed to make you hallucinate and thereby access your unconscious, much in the same way as using hallucinogenic drugs might. The benefit of breathwork is that the effects will disappear as soon as you change your breath, which isn't the case with LSD, ayahuasca or psilocybin. With those, once ingested, you're in for the long haul, like it or not.

I started laughing. Super hilarious giggles. On my own, laughing at my own private joke, whatever it was. There was no joke, nothing going on in my head, just the urge to laugh, so laugh I did.

The thing about the breathing method we were doing is that it puts you in a kind of slightly dreamlike state, even though you are totally aware of where you are and who you are. I felt less inhibited than I might normally be about making noise – laughing maniacally, in this case – in a room with four strangers.

After the laughing stopped, I did some more breathing and listened to the music playing. Maybe laughing was all that was going to happen. That was okay. I remembered the one time I had taken LSD as a teenager and spent the first hour laughing uncontrollably. It definitely beat the following 15 hours of frantically trying not to spiral into a mental re-run of *Poltergeist*-meets-*The Exorcist*.[3]

But then a wave of sadness washed over me, and I felt the familiar tension of tears clench my throat. Agh, REALLY? I was going to cry. I came out of the breathing for a bit to try to regain control, but Matthew knelt down next to me and reminded me to breathe.

Fuck. Fuck. Fuck. I was going to bawl. I could feel it rising. I let it go and surrendered to the experience. Why was I crying? Was I *that* suggestible to emotive music?

I was still sad about losing my mum. I felt the wounded child inside me crying out for security. I missed her; I mourned my childhood. When you lose your parents, or the parent that was there in your childhood, you lose your childhood, which I didn't realize until it happened to me. You lose the person – or people – who can recount to you the funny times, the first words, the birthdays, the pets and the Christmases.

Losing Christmas was a big thing for me. It's still a big thing. I'm welling up as I'm writing this, feeling the ache in my chest for those beautiful, perfect days, what seemed like the one day of the year when Mum would let go and have fun, when she wouldn't work. She was always working, every day, and often into the night. Working to keep everything going. To keep that roof over our heads. Christmas felt like the one day I had her to myself.

I know that wasn't literally true. But that was the emotion that came whooshing up from my belly and through my heart.

---

[3] I've concluded that I've got way too dark an imagination to be good at hallucinogenic drugs. Bloody love a painkiller though.

Matthew gave me a cushion to hug. "Do you have children?" He asked in a low voice. I nodded, sobbing. "Hug the pillow like you'd hug them. Comfort yourself like you'd comfort your own child," he added. "And breathe. Six breaths and this is over. It's gone. You won't hold it anymore." He helped me breathe. Six deep, intense breaths. I breathed the loss in and out. Terrible, deep loss I already thought I'd dealt with. But it was still there.

The healing journey is a spiral. Around and around, past the same points, coming back to them to look at them from different angles, to heal in different ways. A spiral, starting at the centre, radiating out into peace.

The feeling ebbed away. I slowed my breathing for a bit. Matthew tapped me on the shoulder. "Well done," he whispered, and left my side.

I got back into the breath and listened to the music. And it was exactly as though my brain – or my emotional system – was saying, *okay, great, we're doing this, huh, okay here's another one for ya, Anna.* Like, throwing boxes out of that Indiana Jones hangar one after the other, gleeful that finally I was allowing some space to be made. Eminem was now playing, and that opened up all the angry feelings I had about one particular topic, which were pretty close to the surface, courtesy of Toxic Masculine Carl.

Now, I would like to reiterate here that I bear no ill will at all against Carl – I don't know the man. I spent one breathwork workshop in his presence, and never saw him again. In fact, I have a lot of sympathy for him. No, we weren't likely to be friends, but he'd been in the military in war zones and I can only imagine the terrible things he saw. I one hundred per cent believe that Carl was presented to me as an opportunity by the universe to focus me on my rage toward the toxic masculine in our society, and God bless the universe, because it worked.

I felt waves rush up through me of the kind of anger that you get when someone has just done a really incendiary, dickish thing and you almost laugh because it's SO bad that something ticks off in your brain, saying YES. YES, you are FULLY PERMITTED to blow up about this. BLOW UP, MY FRIEND. GO FOR IT.

You know these are the few lulling seconds before you retaliate in a pure, perfect, unadulterated rush of annihilation.

I'm saying this like you can all relate to this feeling. Perhaps you can't. We all feel in different ways for sure. For me, this atomic-level fury gets unleashed roughly every five years. It's rare, but when it happens, you need to run.

I am a person that doesn't like being angry. I'll get irritated and roll my eyes all the time, but that's not anger. That's mild irritation, and usually after a glass of wine and a good meal and maybe (if it's bad) a bath and a vent to a friend, I'm good – that, or I'll just hang on to it and brood on it for a few years until I AM really mad about it. I don't like being angry, and I usually protect my precious calm at all costs. Calm is everything to me. I hate stress and stressy people or situations.

Yet that moment where you tick over into a kind of sublime fury… there's something amazing about that feeling, right? You know it's coming. You know you can't stop it. Like a sneeze or an orgasm. You know you're going to say everything that's been bothering you for the past five years. And it feels GOOD.

Women are not good at expressing anger. We are trained not to be angry. Women are expected to be pleasant and amenable (again, I refer you to the experience of being told to smile in the street). Even in our breathwork session, Matthew and Adam had talked about this being the case in their experience with breathwork. They saw plenty of women who would scream, shout and curse during a breathwork session, releasing the held-in anger. They also saw plenty of women who found it hard to let go and release it. The conditioning runs deep.

I felt the anger welling up in me. I was angry at men. I was angry at all the times I'd been frightened to walk home alone. The times that total strangers felt it was okay to catcall me, shout at me, lean out of cars, yell at and harass me. And about women being murdered while jogging or walking through parks. I was also still furious about the crapness of female healthcare. About, generally, how women's bodies seemed to be considered fair game for neglect and abuse.

But more than that, I was heartbroken about all the women who had suffered far more than me. I was furious on their behalf. A phrase bubbled up within me. I imagined standing in front of a group of women, holding a baseball bat. *If you want them, you'll have to get through me first.* I murmured the phrase, experiencing the truth of that feeling. I felt violently protective of those women. Girls. Children. I was so fucking angry at men who had hurt them, threatened them, killed them. I wasn't angry with Carl. I was angry with the world that would allow this to happen.

Matthew and Adam had both appeared at my side now. I was crying but furious. "What do you want to say? Say the words," Matthew said in a low voice. I tried to say them, but I felt ridiculous. "Say it!" they urged. "Tell them. Tell those bastards. Say it now, then it's done."

I can't remember exactly what I said, but it was along the lines of, *You think you know about pain, you don't know fucking anything, don't you dare hurt them, if you want them you can go through me first, you fucking c**ts.*

You know, something nice and normal like that.

Totally normal to be shouting that in front of strangers, above the mechanics workshop, on the industrial estate, by the canal. I'm now imagining a flock of swans taking off from the surface of the water in indignant fright at the sound of my swearing filling the air.

I slumped back onto my mat. I'd been sitting up, grasping both men's hands hard as I screamed that out. Like an anger birth. *Congratulations, Anna, it's a c-word!*

I lay there, panting, feeling an almighty headache bloom in my brain. "Good work! Take the breathing back to normal now, everyone," Adam said, turning the music down and the lights back up.

We had ten minutes to re-centre ourselves, have a cup of tea and a biscuit (of course), and come back together for a debrief.

I was exhausted. Yet, strangely, once I came back to normal, there was no trace of the emotions that I'd just been riding – a little like my intense emotions during past life regression that disappeared as soon as I "came back". I felt composed and normal, apart from my headache, which took two days to go. I took that as a sign of my outgoing trauma making its mark.

We talked about our experiences openly. I was surprised to find that my two fellow participants had also undergone some intense journeys of their own. They'd been in the same room as me, but I'd been totally unaware of them. The breathwork was like a waking dream.

"You've done some great work today," Matthew and Adam told us. "Go away, rest up, drink plenty of water. Let the healing work now." We left the womb-like room filled with its cushions and soft lights and crystals and tea, and entered the normal world again.

Carl's car wouldn't start. A little gift from the universe.

I'd like to reflect for a moment here on the unusual nature of my breathwork session before telling you how it moved my life along in a quite pivotal way. I value my three hours with Matthew and Adam for a variety of reasons (at the point of writing, I haven't been able to go back for more sessions because of Covid, but I will), not least the profound and intense healing that they facilitated. But also because Matthew and Adam are not hipsters. They are not topknot guys. I'm not anti-hipsters at all, but maybe that's the type you're imagining as I describe all this. They are two ex-roofers. Blue-collar men who had spiritual revelations (see Matthew's story as follows) in the most mundane of situations and changed their lives totally to be in service to healing.

If you want to talk about gifts from the universe, I am grateful to have received the gift of Matthew and Adam holding my hands and spurring me on as I screamed out the fury I had for misogyny in the world. In all the world, here were the ones who facilitated that specific healing for me. Two men from the demographic that, perhaps, at one time or another, I might have thought of as toxic or uninformed or aggressive. That seems meaningful to me.

In the months afterwards I felt so much lighter. I had finally let go of so much trauma I was hanging on to – a lot that I wasn't aware of. Just one session had worked wonders for me. I had several realizations. One was that I was still angry about the whole worldwide situation of domestic abuse/rape/murder/harassment of women and children, but now I was angry about it in a more calm and centred way, rather than the plate-throwing rage of before. That had actually made me feel panicked and less able to think about what I could do in a real way to make positive change (contribute to charities, support people in the front line).

As I had cleared some space in my unconscious by doing this healing, I was able to focus much more objectively on my finances and set plans and goals to make more money. I was able to re-imagine myself as a person who was good with money, who had money and in fact loved money. I manifested more money and opportunities from my writing work. I learnt better and more effective ways to manifest what I wanted in my life.

Another important thing I realized: the more we heal, and the more boxes we can throw out of the hangar, the better our powers of manifestation and magic are. I had a reading one day with Tiffany, my psychic and healer friend, who said, "Spirit wants me to give you an image. It's the infinity sign. The eight on its side. They say, see it flowing from one side to the other. One side is your magical life, one side if your normal life. You are the point in the middle. They are saying, don't forget that both sides are in the other. They're saying, stay balanced in the middle and let more of your magical life into your home life. Your real life. It's all real. That's the message."

From that image of the infinity sign, or lemniscate, came my realization about the relationship between healing and magic. If magic is the art of causing change in accordance with your will[4] (you might prefer to call this "manifestation") then

---

[4]   Although, knowing what your true will is isn't that straightforward, according to some.

you can see that as an active principle. Magic is something you do in the world to change your experience of the world (note that I said, "to change your experience of it", rather than "to change it itself". Some might argue that as we create our own reality, we are the world, and the world is us). Healing fulfils the more passive (though effort-full!) arc of the lemniscate: letting go. We let go. We release. Like trees in autumn and winter, we shed our leaves. In spring, we grow them again (make something new: magic).

In reality, both sides of the shape are magic – the letting go and the making, the dark and the light, the active times and the reflective times. The washing-up and the magic circles. The laundry and the candle-burning. The groceries and the incense. The healing and the manifestation.

I also genuinely feel that because that one breathwork session allowed me to lay aside some heavy emotional burdens, I was able to make meaningful changes to my physical health. Engaging in my emotional healing has always been an act of self-love, and now I was going to take that self-love to the next level.

Yes, I was going to undergo painful, disruptive surgery. Hurrah! Let the self-love begin!

Interview with Matthew Donnachie, Breathwork Practitioner

What is breathwork?

I see breathwork as a rapid trauma-release tool. It's something we used thousands of years ago. Very often with these healing modalities we tend to think they're new, but in fact it's only really that we stopped using tools like that at some point, and started looking at mental health in a different way. For a long time we had forgotten tools like breathwork whereby we can effectively and appropriately process deep emotions.

In recent times, society has taught us that emotions aren't acceptable and that people should keep them in, suppress them, not show that side of ourselves. We're stuck in our understanding of emotions because we've focused on talking about our emotions, but we can't really process emotions through the mind: it has to be done through the heart, or the feeling part of Self. So, for me, breathwork is the fastest, most effective and graceful way of being able to deal with deep trauma that causes symptoms like depression, anxiety and PTSD. It's really helped me deal with all of those things in a safe way.

How does it work?

The style of breathwork that I use is a breath to get you out of your conscious mind, which you could say represents 10 per cent of your mind, and into the subconscious mind, which is the 90 per cent. It's almost like a different part of Self. The breath keeps the conscious mind busy with a task, so that the person is able to connect with the unconscious. The unconscious knows exactly what you need to do, and the deep, profound healing that needs to happen.

The breath style itself is called a conscious connected breath: breathing through the mouth and concentrating specifically on the in-breath. There's no break in the middle from inhale to exhale, but we regulate the speed of the breath depending on what the client is feeling. It's not a strain to the breath but it's a nice consistent rhythm. When clients connect with an emotion while breathing, we may ask them to speed it up slightly, but what we're not doing is holotropic breathing, which is breathing so fast that you hyperventilate. When a client hits an emotion, the sped-up breathing helps them to push through it, to breathe through the feeling.

However, we also ask clients to slow the breath down sometimes. If you're stuck in fear, anger, guilt or sadness, something like that, once you're aware of what it is, there's no point hanging out with that emotion, so we speed up through it, process it. But if you hit joy or bliss – and those are also emotions that we suppress – then we might slow down the breath and let you stay there and feel that. We don't experience enough joy in our lives, certainly not as much as we did when we were children. In fact, throughout our lives we limit our joy, and so when people do feel joy in breathwork, we want them to feel that so they can know what it is and bring more of it into their lives.

What's it like to have a treatment?

Clients lie down, usually on a treatment table or a mat on the floor with a pillow. You're fully dressed. We play music and get the client to start the breath, and then we're there to support and hold the space for the client. We play the music to help trigger emotions. It isn't necessarily chosen because it's sad or happy; sometimes it can be the words, but I usually choose the songs based on where the person was when they were singing it. So for someone like the performer Adele singing 'Someone Like You', where she was at when she was recording that song was such a place of desperation, that's the vibration that comes through the song. So I use a lot of opera, because it's probably the most extreme of the vibrations in music. It really brings out joy and bliss. I'm not curating the playlist in any particular way but I see it as putting opportunities there for people to feel sad, feel anger, should they need or want to. The beauty of it is that it responds to people's needs. So if you need to feel joy, if you hear a sad song, it's not going to touch you. So, sometimes people say, "How did you know to play that song?" I didn't, it's just that the client reacted to what they needed at the time.

Sometimes I will talk to people as they're processing their emotions or hand them a pillow or hold their hand if they need it, but I keep interventions to a bare minimum. Sometimes you need to give people permission to do what they need to. If they need to shout, shout. If they need to punch a pillow, punch a pillow.

If I start talking to a client during breathwork, there's the risk it will start to engage their conscious mind and thereby bring them out of that healing space. So I guide sometimes by saying things like, "It's safe to feel this now" or "Good job" or "Nothing's right or wrong, it just is," but it's about trying to serve without making it about me, the therapist. It's about creating the space for the client to do what they need to do.

Everyone is different in terms of what they do. Some people need to shout to be heard. Some people don't. If our trauma is based around never being able to speak our truth, then it's good to be able to shout. For other people it might be more about needing to acknowledge it within themselves.

A lot of people that try breathwork have tried a lot of other things first to improve their happiness, but haven't necessarily found it. Often, people are blown away! The reason for that is that it's not often that we have an experience of connecting with what I would call our Higher Self or that larger part of the Self. It can be very otherworldly, like we connected with something we didn't even know existed.

Suddenly discovering that you can be in control of how you feel – that you can change that, regardless of the situation – can be a bit like, "Woah! Why did no one tell me about this before? I never knew stuff like this existed!" People ask, "Why don't we have this in schools?" Like, basically why do adults have to wait all this time to find this very simple tool that changes everything? It's like a homecoming to Self but also a discovery of who you can be. Many people talk about it being a second chance.

How did you come to breathwork?
I experienced a lot of childhood trauma that led to depression and anxiety and a habit of beating myself up mentally. I saw a lot of counsellors and psychologists to try to improve my mental health. Anger was a big issue for me. The root of it was, "Why am I being treated this way?" and I just couldn't find anything that was effective in helping me deal with the emotion underneath. Talk therapies were good at helping me process what had happened but I didn't find anything changed. In terms of anger management, I found the experience of going into someone's office for an hour and them poking you for answers about why you were angry – and then asking for £150, off you

go – just made me angry!

I got to a stage in life where I was so desperate that I would have tried anything! I tried yoga and meditation. They gave me something, but it wasn't the deep, profound healing I needed.

One day, I was standing on a roof working with another builder. My mind was on other things and I hit my thumb for the third time in a minute. In a moment of desperation, I stood there and thought, do I throw myself off the roof or just the hammer?

I figured out in that moment that it wasn't that I wanted to die, but that I just couldn't keep going the way I was.

The builder that was standing next to me looked at me straight in the eye and said, "Would you do anything to change your life?" and I said, "Are you crazy? Of course I would."

Long story short, two hours later I was in my first breathwork session, and from that day, my life changed. I knew that I'd found a tool that could help me get these emotions out of me: something I'd been looking for fifteen years.

How has breathwork changed your life?
I couldn't put my finger on what it was at first but I knew there'd been a fundamental change. After two or three sessions I noticed that my behaviours were changing. Until that point I'd always been telling myself *I'm not good enough*, because of the way that I was treated when I was younger, but that wasn't actually true and I was starting to realize that.

People only treat you the way they feel about themselves. Having an abusive parent doesn't mean you're bad. It just means that unless someone's dealt with their own stuff, they can't treat you any differently from how they treat themselves.

I noticed there weren't as many negative comments within my own mind. So for instance if I went to pick up the newspaper at the shop and they didn't have it, usually there would be some choice swear words, then I'd get into blaming them, get aggressive about it. After a few breathwork sessions it was like I was given the choice about how to react. I saw that I didn't have to be angry. I could walk a hundred metres down the road and get the newspaper somewhere else. Before, there was no way to control that anger; it would just come out and then I'd think, *Oh no, what have I done?* But now there was space in between for me to make that choice.

That came with family as well. As everyone is aware, family knows where those big red buttons are. They knew what to say to get a reaction from me. But again I found there was space between what they said and how I responded. That blew my mind! Before, it would be an instant anger – *I can't believe this, what the f**k do you mean*, you know. Now I was able to stand back and think, *That's interesting.* I could still feel anger and disappointment but I'd also think, *How important is this, really? Not very. Do I really care? No.*

So it gave me a different way to be in the world. I mean, this kind of instant anger reaction is everywhere you go in the world. You get two guys in a pub who are willing to go outside and beat ten bells out of each other because one says the other one looked at him funny! And the chances are you were actually looking at this guy's hair, thinking, that's quite a nice haircut, but then before you know it you're outside fighting and if anyone asked you what happened, you wouldn't know. "He said this, and I just lost it," is all you could say because you don't have the space between you and your emotions.

When I worked in building and construction, nothing ever went my way or worked out, but that was because nothing ever went my way or worked out within myself. Now, I run my own clinic. I'm working with some Harley Street psychologists, I do workshops in schools. I think I've got the best job in the world because I get to help people see who they really are, and there's nothing better than that. I feel as though I was given a second chance and it's such a joy to be able to share that.

CHAPTER 10
A TRIAL BY BLOOD: PART 2

Where were we with the bleeding? I'm sorry, but that part of the story isn't quite done.

Ah, right. So, if you recall, I'd exploded with blood at a local park and terrified some dog walkers, and the GP had put me on two of the evil, soul-destroying norethisterone a day and made a request for an appointment with the NHS gynaecologist.

Taking two norethisterone a day meant that I was barely functioning as a human. I was depressed and felt totally disconnected to life. Everything was grey. I frequently cried just from feeling hopeless. The bleeding was still daily but minimal, a brown sludge. I had frequent urine infections and itching. I was also getting heart palpitations and had high blood pressure. A couple of times, I had chest pains. I'm pretty sure that if I'd stayed on that medication much longer, I might have had some kind of cardiac issue.

I'm telling you all this in detail because I want to be absolutely clear about what women are expected to cope with – by society and by the medical community – as part of their daily reality. I was continuing to work, parent and run my life. I felt less than human, and certainly less womanly than I should.

When I finally got to talk to the NHS gynaecologist (on the phone – Covid times) she was spectacularly unhelpful.

I outlined my medical history and the failure of any medication to stop my excessive bleeding.

"So. You have heavy periods, hmmm?" she asked, disinterestedly.

"No, I have excessive bleeding with no breaks. They're not periods," I answered.

"Okay. Well, we would advise an ablation or a Mirena coil next. Has your doctor talked to you about those?"

"Yes. I don't want them. I want a hysterectomy," I had come prepared to the conversation; I was very clear by now about what I wanted.

"Our procedure is that you have to try one of them – coil or ablation. The Mirena coil has made a huge difference to thousands of women. It's significantly reduced the number of hysterectomies we've had to do in recent years," she explained, sounding exasperated. I'm sure she was tired and overworked – not surprising, given the pandemic.

Incidentally, I'm sure that this fact is true, about the Mirena coil reducing the number of hysterectomies given. If you're refusing to give hysterectomies to women before making them use the Mirena coil for anywhere between six months and a few years, your hysterectomy numbers *will* go down as a result – but that's probably only because the coil, or the ablation, or the other medications I'd tried, are ways to "kick the can down the road" and not treat the root cause of the issue.

Logically, this means that in many cases, women are suffering for longer before finally being offered the only operation that can give them their lives back again. I'm sure also that for some of these women, by the time they've tried the medications, the ablations and the coil, they might have begun the menopause, and that can provide an end to symptoms for many.

Again, I get that we have a stupendous free National Health Service in the UK and I wouldn't ever want it to go away, but what would be great would for it to be properly funded and resourced rather than progressively underfunded for so many years that the doctors and nurses don't have the time to respond quickly to patients' needs in what are deemed "non-urgent" conditions. It would also be great for far more investment in medical research for women's health, so that we have a better choice than either burning off layers of our uterus (which DOESN'T EVEN WORK) or the nuclear option of a physically traumatic surgery, as the only real way for us to get an end to seriously debilitating symptoms.

"Well, we won't put you on the waiting list for a hysterectomy without trying one of those treatments, and the waiting list is currently around two and a half years. Probably longer now, with Covid."

That was the way it was. There was no bypassing the system, it seemed, and after I'd been in for an examination – which would again take months – I might have to wait three years for an operation.

I got off the phone and cried. This was hopeless. It had already been around two and a half years and I really didn't feel that I could cope for another three. Again, it felt like no one would help me, no matter how hard I tried.

I sat and stared at the wall, and felt that familiar Babalon-ish rage fill me. This was ridiculous, and I wasn't going to take it lying down.

I didn't have health insurance – I live in the UK, and we have free healthcare here, which I am eternally grateful for – but as I sat in my chair feeling the rage of Babalon envelop me, I wondered how much it would cost to have the operation done privately, and whether that was even possible. I did a search on my phone. It didn't look like it was possible for me to have it done locally with BUPA, but I looked at other options.

I found a Nuffield private hospital quite near to me, and their helpful website listed different gynaecologists that did operations there.

The second number I called was answered by a very helpful receptionist who listened to what I had to say and booked me in for a phone chat within a week with Dr Kent, who, she assured me, was excellent. "He's done a few bits for me, and

THE PATH TO HEALING IS A SPIRAL

he was brilliant," she confided in me. "That's actually how we met – I'm his wife."

I thought it was probably a good sign that Dr Kent was confident enough in his work to have married one of his gynaecology patients, so I paid £200 in advance of our phone consultation. As I was still working and didn't have to commute into the office, which was actually quite expensive for me, I was saving about £400 a month in lockdown, what with also not going out or doing anything.

When I spoke to Dr Kent a week later – just a week! – he couldn't have been more helpful or knowledgeable. I told him that the NHS doctor had wanted me to have an ablation or the Mirena coil. He said, in his experience, neither was very effective, and it sounded like they'd both be pointless for me. He booked me in for an examination a few weeks later and said that he suspected I possibly had a combination of endometriosis and a complication with scarring from my caesarean section all those years ago. He said, if he was right, he'd be more than happy to perform a hysterectomy.

A few weeks later I went along to my appointment, nervous about the fact that I was a) going to a hospital in the peak of a global pandemic and b) about to have a pretty invasive internal examination. But I kept reminding myself that this had to be done, and, furthermore, that this was an act of self-love. I was doing this for myself because I desperately needed it, and I'd damn well find the money if I needed the operation.[1]

In person, Dr Kent was one of those incredibly posh and brisk male doctors, but he was also kind and sympathetic – and, most importantly, he knew his subject. For the first time, I actually felt understood and heard, and I learnt a lot. He, with the help of two nurses, got me into a chair, feet in stirrups, turned me head down and feet in the air and got a camera inside my uterus.

---

[1]   For transparency, I had my hysterectomy with Nuffield, who I couldn't recommend highly enough. The private examination fee was £1,000, and the operation itself including everything was £8,000. I got a loan out for the money and it was genuinely the best £9,000 I've ever spent.

It was a mortifying and certainly less than dignified process, but they did their best, as doctors and nurses always do, to be as nice as possible about it. Again, the sheer grace and nobility of medical professionals humbled me.

I'd like to labour the point that at this juncture I had been suffering with excessive bleeding for around three years, and this was the first time that a gynaecologist had given me a proper examination. And I'd had to pay to get it.

It was exactly as he'd thought. I had a scar in my uterus from my C-section which, having been done in an emergency, probably hadn't been done as carefully as it might have, and had healed badly. There was endometriosis in the scarring, which was causing the bleeding. I also had polycystic ovary syndrome (PCOS), which wasn't helping. Dr Kent explained that this wasn't that unusual and only a hysterectomy would solve the issue – and he was happy to do the surgery for me. I'd have to speak to his wife to book it in and he apologized because it would probably be about six weeks before he could do it.

Six weeks.

Yes please!

In October 2020, as the pandemic raged around us all, I had a hysterectomy, and it was one of the best choices I've ever made.

It was a scary choice, don't get me wrong. I was terrified of going into hospital. I was by now phobic about hospitals because of all my negative experiences in them: watching my mum die in pain and confusion, long stays with her before then for cancer treatment, my own emergency C-section with my son, the weeks I was in hospital with him for suspected meningitis when he was a baby. Never mind the fact that I'd have to go to hospital during a pandemic, even though the hospital I was going to had remained free of Covid cases. I would have to go on my own, unaccompanied. I wasn't allowed visitors. No one was. I had to do it alone.

Fortunately, I had a number of my healing techniques to help me deal with all this fear. One of the things I did was send reiki ahead of me to the hospital when I went in to have my examination and for the surgery itself. One of the four reiki symbols enables practitioners to send the healing to places and future occurrences (and to heal the past, also) so that you can create a positive, healing environment for yourself. You can be creative about it and send it to find specific things for you, like good parking spaces and welcoming people, and ask it to help with things like dispersing traffic and making sure your train runs on time. Honestly, the only thing you're limited by is imagination.

Anyway, I sent reiki ahead of myself to ensure that everything would run smoothly for the operation, that it would be a healing and calm environment. I also asked for help from my various magic and healing groups and I know that they sent me healing and power. I also asked my Reiki Master Gillian to send healing.

I was still nervous going in, but I also knew that I was riding a huge wave of high vibrational energy.

What did I learn from this experience? I learnt that, sometimes, healing involves surgery.

It might seem, in this book, that I hate doctors and conventional medicine. Not at all – in fact, I love anything that works. I'm a results-focused person when it comes to health. *Did it work? Did it help?* That's what I want to know. The reason I love reiki so much – and BodyTalk and breathwork – is because they worked for me. They weren't funny little theories that people can believe in if they're especially credulous. They work, even if you don't understand why.

My hysterectomy worked. But there have been many times in my life when conventional medicine didn't seem to work. Or, more specifically, the humans in those communities were not helpful, perhaps because attitudes to women's health need some improvement. So, I am not anti-doctors, or nurses. I'm anti the current bias in medicine to under-research gynaecology, and I'm anti a progressively underfunded NHS.

For the record, I love nurses. Nurses have never been anything but lovely every time I've had to see one.

Nurses are like gods to me. I can't imagine how they do their job and manage to be amazingly caring and fantastic every day.

That goes for the improbably named Nurse Audrey Hepburn, the real-life, non-film-star nurse with a film-star name that taught me how to breastfeed (you wouldn't forget that name). Here's to the nurses that have cheerfully done my cervical smear tests over the years, the nurses that looked after my mum when she was dying, the nurses that brought me cups of tea and helped me walked to the toilet after my hysterectomy, that made being naked and vulnerable and in pain less embarrassing.

So, for me, surgery worked. And I am so, so happy I did it.

I was really scared of having a general anaesthetic. I'd never had one before and I was plagued with thoughts about those horror stories I'd read about people being awake during surgery and unable to let anyone know that they could see, hear and feel everything.

I didn't sleep the night before the operation. I was just too nervous. The hospital had provided me with some antibacterial soap sponges to use in the shower the night before and the morning of the operation, and I'd shielded as best I could for the weeks before the operation, but I was paranoid that I had somehow picked up Covid and wouldn't be allowed to have it.

Thankfully, I was allowed in the hospital and had passed all my tests a couple of days before. Now, all I had to do was let it happen. As Debbie Reynolds says in the movie *Halloweentown*: "Magic is very simple. All you have to do is want something and then let yourself have it."

I arrived at the hospital early on a Saturday morning, in a taxi, on my own. I didn't know what to expect. I was checked in by a kind receptionist. I was still trying to control my almost vomit-inducing fear of hospitals.

A nurse came and got me from reception – where I had a very pleasant cup of coffee – and took me to my private room. A private room! It was beautiful. Like a hospital that thought it was a Premier Inn. I had my own ensuite bathroom. There was a full menu on the bed. And when I say menu, I mean ten choices for breakfast – pastries, bircher muesli, fruit, eggs benedict – ten for lunch and ten for dinner, plus desserts. I sat on the bed. I was still nervous as hell, but it was also very peaceful up here. Everything smelt nice. There was no chaotic screaming.

I was only there about an hour before I got taken into surgery, and in that time I didn't have much opportunity to work myself up into a lather because Dr Kent came in and explained the operation, a physiotherapist came in and talked to me about pelvic floor exercises to do after surgery, and the anaesthesiologist came in and asked me lots of questions, heartily reassuring me that he would make absolutely sure I wasn't awake during the operation. To be honest, I still didn't believe him, but I was doing this now and there was no going back. I'd taken my knickers off and I was wearing support stockings. This was it.

Two very lovely nurses wheeled me down to a kind of anteroom outside the operating room, and the jolly anaesthesiologist reappeared and stuck a needle in the back of my hand and a mask over my face. I massively appreciated not being shown the inside of the operating room. I know that sounds weird, but I didn't want to see it. I imagined the operating instruments laid out on tables like torture devices belonging to James Bond villains.

That's the last thing I remember until I woke up in the recovery room. I remember absolutely nothing. Nothing at all. A literal blackness. Like being turned off at the mains. It was amazing. I'd done it.

I was wheeled back to my room. I felt euphoric. This was because I had just been given some additional painkillers, and had an oxygen tube up my nose. Let me tell you that oxygen in those quantities is TREMENDOUS. I was so happy. I was also pretty sleepy still, so the nurses kept coming in to check on me, but I was blearily watching *King Kong* with Jack Black when I wasn't snoozing. At some point, a nurse asked if I wanted a cup of tea. I asked if I could have coffee. She said, *sure!* I expected a mug of instant coffee, but I got a cafetière of really nice filter coffee and some cookies. This was shortly followed by the dinner

I'd ordered earlier – stir-fried pork with peppers and couscous, and a lemon posset. Both were delicious.

I was, unexpectedly, having a brilliant time in hospital. It was a hugely privileged thing to do, I know that – I know that many people can't afford private healthcare. I can't, really, but it was incredibly worth it to me to be able to have the operation I needed when I needed it. The fact that I ended up having it in a beautifully peaceful private hospital with an amazing menu was an unexpected bonus. I had taken my health into my own hands, pushed for what I knew I needed and got it, despite the fact that it was scary, it was expensive and there was a global pandemic happening.

I decided that was what was going to happen, and I got out of my own way enough to let it happen.

Before the operation, I had joined another Facebook support group, this time for hysterectomy.[2] This group has been amazing for me in learning more about why people have hysterectomies, the different types you can have (my ovaries were left in, but some people have them out, which causes immediate menopause) and the different recovery times. It also gave me an insight into the potential dangers and difficulties associated with the operation. Recovery was plain sailing for some, not so much for others. There can be complications, depending on everything from pre-existing conditions to how quickly you feel compelled to start doing the housework afterwards (note: the answer to this is, ideally, never doing it again, but as no one wants to live in a hovel, at least five weeks before you hoover. AT LEAST).

Being a part of the group also gave me an opportunity to support other women (including trans men who were having the op too) and share my positive experience. Yet again, it proved to me that women are incredibly supportive of each other, be it in the ladies' bathroom at a club (no one is more supportive than the drunk girls you meet there), the maternity ward, or a group for those who have had hysterectomies.

---

2   What can I say? I'm a big fan of online specialized support groups.

It made me feel less bad for the times before the operation that I wondered whether I should have it. Over and over again, I've seen posts in that group from women who have their operation date booked, are experiencing terrible symptoms – tumours and fibroids the size of footballs making them appear permanently pregnant, agonizing pain from endometriosis, excessive bleeding – but are still questioning whether they should have the operation.

It's a scary operation to have, especially when you've read other women's accounts of what can go wrong afterwards. The recovery time is considerable. Women worry if their families will be able to cope while they're laid up in bed for the standard four to six weeks, never mind the months afterwards as your body slowly returns to normal strength. Who will do the laundry, cook the meals, take the kids to school and football practice and play dates?

Some women were concerned about how long their husbands or partners would "have to wait" until they could be cleared for sex again, which is usually six weeks or so, though it varies and you don't want to rush these things, not least because prolapse is a definite possibility after hysterectomy. (For the unaware, prolapse means that, without your uterus and cervix in their normal places, there are just a few stitches between the sewn-up top of your vagina and your intestines. If the stitches break, or the top of the vagina separates, your intestines will fall into your vagina.)

Leaving aside for a moment being appalled at the male partners who hassle women for sex DAYS after their operations, who moan about the housework not being done, who look after their partners diligently for a week and then start getting passive-aggressive about them being "lazy" – and sadly there are many of these men (as well as plenty of lovely partners who look after their partners for as long as they need it) – there are so many reasons that any of us can get in our own way when it comes to making scary but worthwhile choices in our lives.

Magic is very simple – all you've got to do is want something and let yourself have it.

If we consider "magic" as manifesting what you want in your life – better jobs, more money, love, improved health – the act of creating change in accordance with your true will and in harmony with the universe, then this definition says it all.[3] With the hysterectomy, I and the thousands of women booked in for their operations have the opportunity to let ourselves finally have good health again. It's human to think *better the devil you know*, but if you are ever in a similar situation, if it's scary, if you don't know how you're going to make it work, still let yourself have what you truly want or need.

I was one of the fortunate ones who had no other conditions apart from my defective uterus, and had my husband to look after my son and me until I was shakily able to get up and start getting back to normal. Plus, I could give myself reiki every day. I had six weeks off work, and even after that, I had to take it pretty slowly. By now, this was late 2020 and in the UK we were still under a lockdown, so fortunately I didn't have to commute to my job and could work from home (in my case, my bed). Even after six weeks of mostly lying down, I don't think I could have hacked taking the train into London every day and sitting at a work desk. My abdominal muscles were very weak, I was still sore and got tired easily.

In terms of recovery from hysterectomy, my timeline was roughly as follows:

1–10 hours post-operation: feel fantastic (still have oxygen tube; delicious hospital food; catheter; hospital-grade painkillers). Life is great. Message everyone I know, including some work contacts who are no doubt surprised to hear from me at 11pm. Watch *King Kong*. Consider moving in to the hospital where Debbie and Emma will look after me forever.

---

[3]   This is not the only definition of magic. You can also consider magic as the practice of connecting to deities in a devotional way, magic as a structured way of connecting to other "supernatural" beings to gain knowledge and inspiration from and of them, and magic as a practice connecting yourself to your True Will and ultimately to God. That is a very, very tiny nutshell.

Day after operation, part 1, still in hospital: time to go home! Prove you can walk to the toilet yourself. Think you might die. Pain roughly similar to being forced to climb into a bath by relentless nurse after C-section. Reflect that at least this time I am not required to breastfeed. Husband arrives to drive me home; takes a few fast corners until I inform him he will die a savage, painful death if he doesn't slow down and avoid every bump in the road.

Day after operation, part 2, home: walk up the stairs to bed. Like climbing Everest. Abdomen is filled with knives. Reminded of the story of the Little Mermaid whose every step on dry land was like walking on broken glass. Like the Little Mermaid, seriously regret doing something so stupid to myself.

Day after operation, part 3: cry, get settled in bed, but then have to get up every 30 minutes to wee because nurse has told me to drink gallons of water. Call hospital to ask if the pain is normal. Hospital assures me that it is.

Evening: sleep sitting up in bed as there is no way to lie down. Take Milk of Magnesia and feel like an old person. What is Milk of Magnesia for anyway? Obey surgeon and take it as he has been a genius so far.

Day 2: feel 50 per cent better on waking. Figure out way to lie down. Dose up on painkillers. Sleep. Shower. Sleep. Eat soup. Milk of Magnesia seems to get rid of wind. Excellent. Do some reiki on myself. Feel much better.

Day 4: manage to have a poo. Dear Diary moment. Feel Milk of Magnesia has something to do with it, or the bags of nuts and dried fruit bars I've been eating.

Week 2: follow advice to start walking. Walk from bed to the end of the hall and back again. Do this once a day. Pain when moving slightly less excruciating. Sleep. Daily reiki for about half an hour, and programme it to continue in my sleep.

Week 3: prescribed pain meds run out. Okay on over-the-counter pain meds as long as I don't move. Binge watch Netflix. Sleep. Make it up and down the stairs once to supervise husband making spaghetti bolognese. Stairs now a small hill as opposed to knife-filled Everest.

Week 4: binge watch Netflix. Feel well enough to hold Halloween tea party for son and best friend. Go to bed at 8pm, exhausted.

Week 6: back to work! Can sit up in bed with laptop and work for two-hour bursts before needing a lie down. Everyone on Zoom sees what my bedroom is like. Technically cleared for sex. NO WAY, BUSTER. Like Melissa McCarthy says in one of her movies, it's like a haunted fairground ride down there right now. Be scared of it. Respect it. Do some magical classes online in my pyjamas.

3 months: feel more normal. Go on a proper walk. Okay as long as I have a sit down halfway. Give sex a try. Everything seems to work. Phew.

6 months: try a bit of yoga. Still uncomfortable lying on one side in bed. Still get more tired than usual, but also loving never having a period EVER AGAIN.

12 months: back to proper yoga; feel normal. Utter joy at not being on hormone medication. Feel clear-headed. Wear thongs and white clothes with impunity. This is what being a man must be like.

So let's get back to Babalon here. The goddess Babalon is many things, and She is a deeply complex, spiritual concept that goes above and beyond bleeding and hysterectomies and bodies. To remind ourselves, She is the acceptance of all things, of all existence and reality, the good and the bad. She is the totality of everything and the annihilation of everything. People who believe in the system of Thelema, Aleister Crowley's philosophical-magical system, consider Babalon to be the spiritual state of everything and nothingness that one can only access after death.

Yet the Babalon *current*, as some people call it, is a power – an empowerment – we can all tap into. By "current" I mean an energy present in the world; a kind of frequency that is available for us to tune into, should we feel so inclined.

Babalon as an energy feels rooted in justice and healing for many. Something in that combination of acceptance and love of all, regardless of our transitory human moralities and beliefs about the inherent "goodness" or "badness", is an empowering force. The justice is in the balancing of all things and the loving of all things. At the micro level, for an individual, that very well may mean an acknowledgement that your body is to be loved and valued as much as anyone else's.

I interpret Her energy as also being about acceptance: if we love something fully, we accept it fully. Loving and fully accepting the vile things your body is doing is not an easy task. We are predisposed to value wellness, ease and lack of pain above disease, pain and stress. Yet, ironically, in embracing acceptance of something that is difficult – sitting with it in the here and now, rather than ignoring it – we reduce its power to harm us.

That is why She's relevant in my journey, I think.

Post-hysterectomy, I wonder whether I'm now free of the mother wound. Had I held the trauma of losing my own mother and the trauma of the early years of being a mother myself in my womb? It's possible. For sure, I feel a sense of peace now that I never had before, and I think only some of that is connected to not taking horrible hormone drugs that definitely disagreed with me. I have speculated a few times since having the surgery that maybe that mother wound trauma was removed with my uterus.

If so, EXCELLENT. I don't miss it.

Otherwise, I've given myself a ton of reiki and had some BodyTalk sessions since the hysterectomy, all of which have helped me integrate the experience. As well as having valued therapists I can rely on, it's important to me that I also have the skills to heal myself, protect myself psychically and generally have some STUFF I can do when I need it.

They say knowledge is power, but healing is power too.

CHAPTER 11

TALKING TO THE ANGELS IN LOCKDOWN: ANGELIC HEALING OR "MAYBE ALL THIS LOVE AND LIGHT STUFF ISN'T SO BAD AFTER ALL"

When the lockdown hit in March 2020, initially I thought, like most of us, that I'd probably be home for a few weeks and then it would all get sorted. Back to the office, back to real life.

Clearly, that didn't happen.

After a couple of months had passed, and as the lockdown didn't show any signs of easing, I joined a WhatsApp group my friend Tiffany had started. Seemed like something to do.

In fact, I hadn't been put on furlough, so I was busy working at home at my office job, with book deadlines coming out my ears and a child to homeschool, so I wasn't someone who had a lot of extra time during the lockdown. I had far less time than usual, not least because of having to stop what I was doing every two hours or less and make everyone lunch, attempt some homeschooling, go out for our daily walk or keep up with the mountains of dirty dishes that were now being created because we were all stuck inside. I know many of you reading this will have done the same, and I sympathize with anyone who wanted to do a murder at about Day 16.

Totally acceptable.

Therefore, when Tiffany began her little group, it was perfect, because it was all about spending five or ten minutes a day doing something, and five or ten minutes was all I had.

We began with a thankfulness practice, which I was dubious about, but I knew Tiffany and trusted that she knew what she was on about.

Thankfulness, if you haven't come across it under a broadly spiritual lens, is the idea that you practice being grateful for as many things as you can throughout your day. You say "thank you", out loud, or in your mind, for everything – for the air you breathe, your toast for breakfast, the water in your shower and the job you have, etc.

You also practice being thankful for the things you're not overly thrilled about, like being in a global pandemic and confined to your house doing the aforesaid dishes (I was thankful for the dishwasher, among other household innovations). The more thank-yous you can do a day, the better your powers of manifestation will be, perhaps because it's another way to lavish pleasure and approval on everything *just as it is*, like Mark D'Arcy loves Bridget Jones, creating a psychological shift in your brain. This leads away from dissatisfaction and toward acceptance, like a reprogramming, if you will.

Tiffany taught us that different emotions cause us to "vibrate" at different levels. We all "vibrate energetically" at different levels. I know this is something that most of us can feel when we are in the presence of others, and it can also be contagious. Think of the classic "energy vampire" you may have met who saps your good mood when you're around them, or think of times when you've walked into a party or a room of people and been caught up in a joyful, fun vibe.

According to Tiffany, the higher we vibrate, the easier it is to manifest and make our dreams come true. You can find diagrams online that show you what emotion vibrates at what frequency; I'm not sure that the numbers are that important (while also being aware I'm happy to be wrong about that) but Enlightenment and Peace are right at the top, with Joy and Love right underneath them. For contrast, Apathy, Guilt and Shame are at the bottom. I can't even see Fear on the chart but I'm assuming that's one of the worst offenders.

We would often have a focus for the day to vibrate the emotion of Love, Joy or Peace as much as possible, thereby lifting our vibration and making it easier to visualize the changes we might want to make in our lives. This would be a matter of thinking ten loving thoughts per day – remembering moments that were full of love, thinking of people we loved, parties, loving our pets, whatever.

Just a few minutes every day doing this kind of practice, whether consciously taking some time to feel love or saying thank you for everything you can think of in your life, actually did make a huge difference to my daily wellbeing. Like a kind of focused meditation, it was a way to feel like you were doing something good and worthwhile every day in lockdown, amid the ridiculous work/meal-making/homeschooling/only-going-out-for-one-prescribed-walk-a-day fiasco.

This whole focus in the group was on creating better conditions for us to manifest our dreams come true, and after practising our thankfulness and vibration-raising, we moved on to angelic healing. Cue more face-pulling from me. After working with "dark" goddesses like The Morrigan and Babalon, doing exhausting primal screaming and the like, I was slightly disparaging about angelic healing. If it wasn't hardcore – that is, if it wasn't all about death, serious magical transformation and war, pain and sex gods – then frankly I didn't feel very into it.

For someone who had been brought up as a kind of mystical Christian, the notion of angels wasn't unfamiliar, but it still felt a bit too woo-woo for my tastes (I know. Pot, kettle, black). It wasn't that I disliked standard Christianity, I just never felt that it was for me. I'd go to our local church with my mum when I was a kid (when Mum was in her Church phase), sit there and listen, and feel completely underwhelmed by the Church of England.[1] There was no magic or mystery to the thing. There was no Latin or incense or tales of death and destruction and the vicar didn't seem like a particularly exemplary or wise person. Such was the harsh assessment of an eight-year-old.[2]

Regardless, here I was on WhatsApp, doing angel meditations – which isn't very Church of England at all. Every day, Tiffany posted little meditations and tasks for us to do, aimed at helping us manifest what we wanted into our lives. Part of this was working with angel energy – the Archangels Michael, Gabriel, Raphael and Uriel – sometimes with gods and goddesses, such as the Buddhist goddess of mercy and compassion Quan Yin, and sometimes those who are called "Ascended Masters", people who have been alive on the earth at one stage but are now spiritual masters or teachers in other realms, for example Jesus, Mary Magdalene and Lord Maitreya.[3]

Typically, with these energies, we would do a short meditation inviting the angel in question to communicate with us and to accept their healing. This would be something along the lines of centring ourselves in a quiet moment and taking notice of our breath and then imagining the presence walking toward us, and visualizing certain details about the angel or god or master, and

---

[1]   If religions were biscuits, in my opinion the Church of England would be a Rich Tea – which, for non-UK residents who might be reading this, is a very boring (but inexplicably popular) biscuit.

[2]   In fact, that same vicar did a successful exorcism of a malignant spirit that was living in our house when I was a kid, so what do I know? Sadly, that's too long a story for this book, but I respect the Church more for it.

[3]   Lord Maitreya is believed by some to also have incarnated as Krishna and was closely associated with Christ in Theosophy. He is also known as Lord of the World and is dedicated to making the world a better place as well as protecting it.

asking for a blessing from them. We would be encouraged to feel the high vibrational energy of the angel or god and bask in it; feel its energy surrounding us and protecting us. Usually we would end by thanking the angel for its presence and imagining putting on a magical cloak of protection afterwards. I always found these meditations powerful and, in the case of the Archangels and the goddess Quan Yin in particular, it led to me calling on their energies when doing reiki sessions with others. I find Quan Yin a deeply compassionate, beautiful energy. Whenever I connect with Her (in meditation, or when giving reiki) it's like a pink aura overcomes me, full of an intense feeling of maternal love.

We also focused on connecting with our own personal guardian angel. Now, this is something that I had done before without really trying to, mostly in dreams. I had always experienced a guardian-angel-type presence as male and roughly resembling a sexy Jesus (don't laugh, I'm SERIOUS) or Duff McKagan, the original bassist from Guns N' Roses.[4] Over the years I've had many dreams with Duff-Jesus where he is teaching me things – a generous-spirited, wise and insanely hot spirit friend. At other times, this energy and visions of this guide have come through when I've had reiki, or when I was attuned to it. There was a time when I was finding things especially difficult – having a kid under three, exhausted, working – when I would imagine Duff-Jesus riding in the car with me when I was driving to and from work. It was a comfort to imagine and feel him with me; we listened to music together and I felt a little less lonely. Is that pathetic? Probably, yes, but it helped.

Again, this guardian angel energy came through to me via Tiffany's various prompts. I felt that same feeling: it's hard to describe, but I sensed the colour yellow strongly, and a positivity, and kind of clean, pure masculinity that felt loving and grounded. It was – and is – there for me when I need it.

We had meditations that asked us to imagine we were sitting in a circle and holding hands. We would imagine that a group of

---

[4] I like 'em tall and blonde, okay?

angels came down from the sky and stood in the middle of the circle. We would call our own guardian angel toward us. They would walk toward us; we smiled as we saw each other; we would hug them, observe their faces, what they looked like. We would feel the love coming from them and listen to any messages they might have for us, and then thank them for their presence.

Connecting to guardian angel energy involved practices like looking for signs – relevant music, images of angels in books and on TV, angel numbers (11:11, 22:22, etc. – there's a lot of information to be found online about these), dreams featuring angels where they appear to you (I had already had those), light orbs, all manner of things. I personally have always felt spirit energy (or angel energy, whatever you want to call it) as feeling like my hair is being brushed from my temples or my neck, or a tickly touch that makes me shiver on my shoulder or on the back or side of my head. So I had this a lot at this time.

Again, there were dreams. Incidentally, it's a good practice to record your dreams as much as you can. This is a common thing in magical training but also good for anyone's mental health, I believe, because it puts you more in contact with your unconscious and what it is trying to tell you. I've found that, over the years, my dream world has developed to the point of having regular locations, people (people who appear in dreams who I don't know in waking life – I presume they are dream guides or spirit guides of some kind) and symbolism that all combines into its own "Anna" world of significance. It makes sense to me but probably wouldn't to others. My dreams will often provide solutions to problems or make me realize something; they often use puns or play with imagery to make a point. If you remember my dreams about the museum of snakes and reptiles, that was pretty literal: it was telling me the only way was through my fears and through the difficult time I was experiencing – like a trip to IKEA, the only way out was through. I had to face up to it all and find a way through it – which I did.

Looking back at my dream journal for the lockdown, I had a lot of dreams about houses (unsurprising, given I and everyone else was inside one for 98 per cent of it), but specifically about a house that had a hidden room, or even a series of hidden rooms that I would discover in my dream.

Often there would be a number of bathrooms that I hadn't known about. There was a sense of rediscovering these rooms, having forgotten they were there. There was also frequently a man in my dreams who kind of showed me around the house, or who I met at other locations such as large, imposing National Trust-type houses, who I knew was magical and would tell me that these houses with the missing rooms were mine and I had to bring those rooms back into operation. Was that my guardian angel telling me that there were elements of my life I was neglecting at that time? That there were parts of myself that I had forgotten? I think it was. With the National Trust-type houses, I think he was showing me just how big my potential power was. He was saying, this is yours, if you want it. If you decide to be mistress of this house, as it were, like a kind of magical Downton Abbey.

In fact, as we all know now, we never returned to "real life" after the lockdown – or, at least, we haven't yet gone back to how it was. Perhaps we never truly will. All of us are changed.

For me, the Covid years (thus far) have represented a huge magical awakening which I don't think would have been possible without a) all the healing I'd done first and b) the kind of isolation, high weirdness and pause from normal life that the pandemic has supplied.

I have been lucky not to have been ill and not to have had to lose anyone close to me at the time of writing. In a way I feel that I've lived my worst years already; certainly the year in which I watched my mum die and then lived – just – through the resulting grief was the worst, closely followed by the first year of my son's life. For me, the pandemic hasn't even come close to those bleak times. As I say, I've been lucky. But I have also treated this time as an opportunity to grow more receptive, more open and pliant to magical training and to trust in my own instinct that this is who I am. This is what I am happiest doing, where I feel I most belong.

In the age of Covid, we are all finding things hard. Many of us have some kind of emotional pain or physical difficulties because of it, and Covid itself is causing and exacerbating a lot of trauma. I hope that this book will help people who are having a terrible time find help, see the world a little differently or feel supported.

The experience of Covid has also taught me a lot about being quiet and receptive and the healing that comes with that. As a society, we are focused on pushing forwards, doing the thing, reaching, working harder. Covid has made us all sit still more. For me it's also opened a world of realization that when I sit back and concentrate on receiving good things, when I enjoy feeling the energy of abundance, the (quite erotic) feeling of receiving all the bounty the universe wants to give me, great things happen.

I adjusted my attitude to work from a kind of fevered chasing of everything, based on fear that it would never happen, to a conscious sitting back and knowing that abundance will come to me. Sure enough, I started being approached for work rather than me chasing it, and extra money started rolling in without me doing anything more than I already had. I think the phrase is "passive income".

During the lockdown, I also improved my daily magical practices. I started using what's called the Lesser Banishing Ritual of the Pentagram more, which is a good grounding and centring meditation used in High Magic, but which would help anyone with focus, clarity and feeling connected to the elements.[5] That led me eventually to join a High Magic[6] group, and from there my magic has improved in leaps and bounds.

---

[5]   You can find videos online showing you how to do it, and I've listed some useful books at the end, too.

[6]   High Magic, or Thelema, uses ceremony and structure in a more fixed way than witchcraft, which, depending on how you do it, can be very instinctive and individual to the practitioner, or more ritualistic. The distinction of "high" magic relates to a more planetary and cosmological approach, whereas "low" magic is more related to the use of the elemental powers of the earth and to the moon (and doesn't mean bad). It also relates to folk magic and that of traditional witchcraft; for example, the older traditions of the cunning folk in the UK.

One of the other things I did in the lockdown was take a few online magic classes, mostly on sigil magic. This was something I already knew how to do, having taught myself, but the classes I took really helped me see what I was doing wrong and how I could improve my practice in that area. *When you're ready, the teacher will appear*, as the saying goes. Well, my teachers appeared, and it seemed that my guides wanted me to learn this particular type of manifestation skill.[7]

Sigil magic is the practice of making a symbol that expresses a particular well-thought-out wish in drawn form. The idea is that the symbol, made correctly, represents the compressed, intense energy of that wish, which you then "release" into the world (I burnt mine, but you can tear them up and release them to the wind, bury them, drop them into the sea, etc.) and into your unconscious as a kind of programme which then allows you to manifest it into reality.

I did a lot of sigil magic in the lockdown (again: why not? Not much else of interest going on) and had an extremely high success rate. For instance, I manifested the precise amount of money within a year to pay off the loan I'd taken to pay for my hysterectomy; I manifested other work that allowed me to pay off a credit card debt; and I manifested a publisher for this book. I also asked for a magical group I could join that would be right for me and a deeper understanding of magic, both of which have happened.

Would I have joined my sigil-making class without feeling empowered enough to do so? Would I have been able to learn these extremely effective manifestation methods without having spent the time clearing out my self-defeating belief patterns that I couldn't or shouldn't do such a weird thing? Definitely not.

Would I feel strong and energetic enough to be able to be an active part of a High Magic group if I was still on norethisterone, bleeding daily? Would I have been able to get fit again with yoga

---

[7]   I have listed a couple of useful books at the end if you would like to look into this very practical technique.

and cycling? No. I don't think I would have. All the meditations, the reiki, the gratefulness practice and breathwork, releasing the witch wound and the mother wound, helped bring me to a place of clarity, without fear and negative self-talk, where I could manifest the life I wanted for myself. I could take control of my own health and wellbeing by making sure I got the surgery I needed – and making sure that I earned the extra money I needed to repay the loan I got to pay for it.

Would I also have been able to remain centred and calm with sometimes quite mansplainy men without having done that deep, intense breathwork healing that helped me heal my relationship with men, the masculine, and dare I say it, the Divine Masculine? Nope.

I wouldn't have been able to write this book without the fortifying, positive techniques of self-belief I learnt from that daily WhatsApp group, and the realizations that came to me while I was reflecting on the experiences of lockdown, quarantine and everything that had happened in my life so far. I wouldn't have written this without that uplevelling of reiki energy that somehow seemed to open doors in my mind – hidden rooms of work potential, transformation of identity, connection to magic and love that my guardian angel wanted to remind me were there, waiting to be inhabited.

Because I pursued healing, my horizons have opened to allow in new possibilities. I've made new projects happen, and one of them is, I hope, this book, which is an attempt at healing at a community level. We need community and generational healing in the wake and aftermath of Covid. We need one-to-one healing for ourselves, and we also need to know and understand how something like Covid affects us and our families in the long term.

I hope that I've gone some way toward explaining, at least, that we all need healing and how we might get it. I also hope that I am starting to make you understand something about the relationship between healing your trauma and your unhelpful, restricting mental and emotional patterning, and causing real and useful change in your life.

Remember – magic (and healing) is very simple. All you have to do is want something and then *let yourself have it.*

It's the *letting ourselves have things* part that trips most of us up.

CHAPTER 12
LOCKDOWN MAGIC

I became a Reiki Master during the 2020–2021 Covid-19 pandemic.

Forgive me, I know that is horribly reminiscent of those irritating guys on Twitter who were saying things at the time like: "If you haven't learned five new languages, got into the best shape of your life and written a novel in the lockdown, you're doing it wrong." I definitely don't mean it that way. It's just what I did.

It was during one of the periods in the lockdown when we were allowed to see people, under restricted guidelines, and it was only really possible because I felt open and positive enough to seek it out and pursue it with Gillian, who I have interviewed earlier in the book. I had found Gillian through a friend some years before but, for whatever reason, I hadn't really pushed myself to follow up Reiki Master training with her.

I say "for whatever reason", but there *was* a reason, which all these healing techniques helped me to push beyond. This is what my mind was telling me before I changed it:

Yes, you like the idea of being a Reiki Master, but it sounds like a lot of work! (It wasn't.)

It's probably expensive. You can't afford that. (It wasn't and I could.)

You're fine as you are! Reiki two works pretty well. (True, I was fine, but Reiki Master energy is waaaaaaaay much more orgasmically, universally WOW and has unlocked plenty of other wow moments in my life.)

You've got other things to think about. (When don't you? Doesn't mean you can't do this, too.)

These are examples of fear-based messages to Self, and they occur all the time. I guarantee you that these types of messages are still knocking around in my brain when it comes to other things in my life that probably need switching up; it's part of being human that our brains second-guess us all the time, to keep us safe.

But, as we've explored, "safe" very often means ignoring the growth you need.

I had an incorrect assumption that Reiki Master-ship was going to be a very long and drawn-out process. In fact, it did take quite a long time because Gillian and I were trying to fit our sessions in between various locked-down periods, which meant that there were months-long gaps between our sessions together. However, it wasn't arduous and it all worked out perfectly.

Typically, what these sessions were like were that I would drive over to Gillian's house, which was about twenty minutes from mine, and park outside a curry house (glamorous location BINGO alert). When I got to her house, we would walk down to the large work room she has at the bottom of her garden and we would have about a four-hour one-to-one session where she would teach me some amazing and far-out knowledge about energy bodies, spiritual beings, extraterrestrials and the possibilities of interdimensional travel.

In true 2020 style, she also performed my Reiki Master attunement in full PPE and a face shield.

Where there's a will, there's a way, and the universe had definitely decided it was time for my Reiki Master attunement to happen. Pandemic be damned!

By the way, for more context, the space which Gillian uses for teaching, gong baths and the like, is chock-full of crystal skulls. Not small ones, either. These are proper *Indiana Jones and the*

Kingdom of the Crystal Skull-type things.[1] She's like a kind of crystal skull herder. Again, from the outside of the house, you would never know this was all going on inside it.

Gillian is a very gentle, quietly spoken, petite grandma with a grey bob. I have never seen her dressed in anything other than sensible slacks, fleeces and jumpers in light blues and greys. I suppose I'm saying this because within the alternative spiritual communities of the world, which are vastly varied and multitudinous, there are lots of people who definitely do dress in certain ways – all the tattoos, all the crystals and beads and spiritual symbols, etc. Again, I'm no stranger to a crystal or a tattoo, to be fair. Sometimes outward image is relevant to what people are doing, or they look a certain way for a clear purpose. But it's also true that healing, magic and power have nothing to do with what you wear or how you look. Particularly with people who practice reiki, I've noticed, in which there is a definite fleece and trainers look.

The Reiki Master attunement itself, despite the PPE and me wearing a face mask, and us having all the windows open in winter so it was fricking COLD, was still as beautiful an experience as the others I had experienced for reiki one and two. In the Reiki Master attunement you are given the final Master symbol to use, and have it "implanted" in your aura, for want of a better phrase.

Each reiki symbol has a certain energy. The Master symbol, from the first time I experienced it, was/is a highly intense and yet gentle rainbow-filled violet-purple energy of interstellar love. That, as twee as it sounds, is how I have experienced it. By that I mean that's how it feels in my body, in the energy fields around my body and when I use it in a treatment for other people.

I remember a previous reiki teacher explaining to me the ways that the different levels feel. I think she said that reiki one is like

---

[1] I know that I constantly reference the Indiana Jones films and I can only put it down to the fact that I'm a child of the 80s and they're great movies! Apart from *The Temple of Doom* which has some dodgy "of its time" misrepresentation of Kali worship.

suddenly realizing that you can run when you've been walking all your life. Reiki two is like driving a car down the street for the first time. Reiki Master is like putting your foot down on the motorway on a beautiful bright morning with a clear road ahead of you and an absolute banger on the radio.

I totally get that now. It. Is. WILD.

Just the other week I did a distance reiki treatment for a friend. In being able to use the Master symbol, the power is ramped up far higher than before and I can really feel that when I am sending healing to someone. On this occasion, it got very hot in the room and I began instinctively doing a type of tantric breathing which increased the intensity even more. We were listening to a playlist of songs themed around Mary Magdalene, and I definitely felt Her energy connect to us as well. It was a very intense, heart-centred feeling of compassion and love: very beautiful and very high vibration.

To explain, when you do a distance healing, you start it in the usual way by requesting that reiki energy be given to whoever it is, and trace the reiki symbols into your hands rather than into someone's energy field in front of you as you would if someone were there. From there, I was taught that you can either visualize a ball of healing light building between your hands and connecting to the person, wherever they are, or you can use something like a pillow or a teddy bear to act as the person and use that as a proxy for them – so, you effectively give the pillow or the teddy reiki, knowing that it translates over to the person. I use both methods. I'm also very instinctive in my treatments, so I will ask for messages from healing guides and obey my instincts as to where to put my hands; if working with a pillow, I might sometimes hug it if I feel that's what the person needs.

After the treatment, my friend described the feeling as "like the last time I took MDMA", which I'm going to take as a compliment (and, for those MDMA lovers out there, maybe give energy healing a go as a non-chemical alternative!). Joking aside, it made sense because MDMA opens the heart centre, or the heart chakra, to give people that sense of love and connection, which is exactly what we were experiencing as part of that healing. Everything was pink; I could see pink energy all around me and (in my mind's eye) all around my friend receiving the energy. Mary Magdalene is also, of course, a goddess figure or Ascended Master associated with love, compassion and magic.

The Reiki Master energy is now always with me, even when I'm not doing treatments or using it in particular ways. Apart from healing oneself and others in hands-on or distance treatments, you can use reiki for almost anything you can think of. Energetic protection of yourself, others, your house, your pets, your car – check. Healing events in the past – check. Healing events in the future – check. Setting up your house so that it's energetically primed to empower you on a daily basis – check. Sending reiki to your office ahead of an important meeting to smooth the way – check. I've also used it to clear traffic jams, find parking spaces, enjoy smooth and uninterrupted train journeys, bring love, new relationships and friendships to me and to heal dynamics in relationships. You can reiki your food and drink to make it extra delicious and good for you, reiki your plants, your garden to make it grow. Cats love it.

The Master energy has also furnished me with a kind of constant lightness and resilience. It's kind of hard to describe, but it's at once the ability to disconnect from stressful situations and the lightness to laugh more, but also the ability to feel more connected to the light skein of being that is the web of all things, with me as an insect-like moving part that skims and flies at speed through the cosmos, rather than a heavy being weighted within its own separateness.

There is a sense of knowing the constant power of the universe that you stand within and can command at any time, relaxed, with no effort – no gyrations, fasting, long rituals or tricky yoga poses required. Don't get me wrong, life is still life, and it continues as it always does. But there is now this knowledge of an even-ness and lightness inside and through it as well, which is best described as the beauty in a single moment of stillness;

the perfection of one breath, and the next. Those still moments of purity stacking up on each other.

In fact, this very book happened as a result of my massively improved manifestation abilities gained during lockdown, of which the Reiki Master attunement and my resulting new energy was a huge part. I had done all this healing (always still more to do, of course) and now I was starting to engage in the other side of the lemniscate: the magic. The "making things happen" part. The strange art of sitting back and letting good fortune come to you while believing it has already happened.

And that, dear reader, is where I am now. Post-lockdown life for me is very different to life at the start of the pandemic, as it probably is for you. Just those two years in themselves have been a huge journey: for me, I lost a uterus and left a day job, gained a lot of new magical knowledge, wrote this book, wrote some other books and remembered who the fuck I am. I realized that healing is even more necessary than it was before, especially in these post-pandemic days. And there are some useful things that I can say about healing, so here they are, I hope.

Please know that healing is there for you. All you have to do is knock, and the door will be opened – and whether it's opened by a middle-aged woman in a fleece and slacks, an ex-roofer or a woman that talks with angels every day, you will find the one that suits you.

CHAPTER 13
A HEALING MANIFESTO AND A NICE CUP OF TEA

It feels like time to start pulling together some of the threads in this book so that we can agree on some kind of healing manifesto, or at least, some principles I've learnt as I've gone along that might help you.

1. We all need healing

I hope, if there is one takeaway for anyone reading this book (and having got all the way to this bit, thanks!) it is this. As humans, we are immersed in this ocean of existence that for all of us will create reasons to need healing. We're all alive. Life is engineered to knock us about a bit. Ergo, we can all heal. There is not one person on Earth who doesn't need it, or at least hasn't needed it once.

2. Anyone can do it

Let go of your expectations that healing is all gong baths with hipsters and aromatherapy massage in Bali. I hope by now I have demonstrated that normal people are doing it every day in very normal, and sometimes completely underwhelming, conditions.

I mean, I don't know if things are different in other countries, but in the UK at least, we have a proud heritage of being distinctly unglamorous, and, in my experience, this has definitely extended to my healing experiences. The healing itself has been far from underwhelming. The locations, the biscuits and the tea, not so much.

You do not need to be a "certain sort of person" – i.e. easily convinced, a bit dim, woo-woo (I hate that phrase but we all know what it means), vegan and wearing handmade clothes (the very idea!) to get healing. It is available to all should you choose it, and it will work for you regardless of whether you "believe" in it or not. Our secularity-obsessed culture has persuaded people that alternative healing techniques are something that one needs to hypnotize oneself in a kind of idiotic haze of credulity to make work. This is simply untrue.

3. You never come to the end of healing

Your stuff is always your stuff, and during the process of healing you may come back to certain issues more than once – hence the title of this book. What happens, though, is that you tend to come back to some of the same issues to heal them *on another level* as time goes by. So that might mean that if you have a big operation, first you heal at the physical level. Then, later, you might come back around to some emotional trauma caused by the surgery or whatever put you in hospital. I certainly had emotional healing to do after my body was technically healed from my C-section. And even after you've been through that once, you might need to come back to it again later. These things can take time.

I've found that this depends on the intensity of the trauma. Some things you can move through pretty quickly. Some things take many attempts. Regardless of where you are in the journey (and everyone's journey is different), I think it's important to remember that the whole thing, like life, is a journey. You could say that life itself was one long healing journey.

On one hand, this is deeply reassuring – we're all in the same boat, and we should let go of the pressure to have "completed" our healing. It's less easy to define than that. No one is handing out badges at the finish line. But there may be opportunities in your life to reduce a load you didn't know you were carrying. That is valuable.

On the other, it's really bloody annoying. It's never done? For fuck's sake.

4. Healing your emotions can be gritty and feelings can be explosive

Yeah, sometimes these things get very *real*. In that room on the industrial estate, I was faced with my own rage and my own sorrow and neither of them were particularly lovely. But it is what it is, as they say.

At the same time, going through a process of healing is never as scary as your mind expects it to be (and therefore invents reasons why you shouldn't do it). Healing the trauma will never be as bad as living through the original trauma. The hard part was living through the trauma in the first place.

Feelings are tricky beasts, in one way, but they're pretty predictable in another. They can easily make us believe things that aren't true, even though they think they're acting in our best interests. Fear often stops us doing things, or tries to stop us. "Feel the fear and do it anyway" is something we've all probably heard, the idea of overriding our mind whose job it is to tell us to avoid things that will upset the applecart. But what if sometimes the applecart is rubbish? What if it *needs* upsetting?

The mind works on a risk-averse "if it ain't broke, don't fix it" model, but is that always enough? In his fascinating book *Thinking, Fast and Slow*, Daniel Kahneman shows us that the hidden, unconscious mind drives most of our decision-making, rather than the conscious, rational mind, as we usually would like to believe. We humans believe we are super rational beings, but Kahneman shows us in a variety of experiments just how governed we are by our desires and emotions.

Mark, my sigil magic teacher, explained it as the unconscious being an elephant, and the conscious mind being a child who sits on the elephant, trying to make it move in a particular direction. Who is in charge in this scenario? It's the elephant, of course. The elephant is much more powerful than the child, and it will pretty much go in the direction it wants to, regardless of what anyone tells it. The elephant/unconscious is full of desire for all the things you would never admit to wanting, but that you do want – sometimes in deeply self-destructive ways. I have listed Mark's book, *The Sigil Secret: Using Magic Symbols to Protect, Heal and Create*, in the list at the end of this book. It's well worth a look.

The conscious mind is the thing "telling" the unconscious what it should do and what it should want, but the unconscious has its own agenda. This is why in "shadow work" as it's currently called (basically just healing), we seek to align the conscious and the unconscious so that they're both pulling in the same direction. Realistically, as the unconscious is much stronger than the conscious – all those deep desires, remember – then it's more logical to make the unconscious conscious, as psychologist Carl Jung said, so that you know what's in there and can love it and integrate it into your life, rather than not knowing, and let it rule your life. I opened this book with a Carl Jung quote:

Until you make the unconscious conscious, it will direct your life and you will call it fate.

That's what it means.

Our minds don't want us to be upset, but they don't always understand (until they've witnessed the process, then they're on board) that sometimes we need to cry and scream and let it all out. Many of us (like me) are the type to bottle up our feelings. Really, I think it's much healthier to be a supercharged and openly emotional person because that way, it all comes out all the time and never has a chance to build up into something really yucky. We all know that when we bottle things up, at some point there's going to be an explosion.

People ask me about healing all the time, but very often, they will rationalize that they don't need it, or that it isn't the right time in their life, or that they just need to find the right modality or time in their busy schedule or what have you.

That's okay. As Maria said in her interview, consent is everything and we must respect whatever journey someone is on. Goodness knows I held on to a lot of emotions for a LONG TIME and avoided the hell out of healing, because it is as scary AF. As they say, you can lead a horse to water, but you can't make it drink.

Our minds will tend to rationalize that we don't need healing, usually until our unconscious takes over and throws a hissy fit of such magnitude that our conscious mind has to sit up and listen. Very often, that hissy fit will involve the unconscious steering us into destructive situations, based on what it wants as a result of an experience somewhere along the line. Matthew found breathwork after his unconscious gave him a sudden urge to jump off the roof he stood on. Gillian found reiki after a rough time with her daughter's eczema. Sometimes (but not always) an extreme event – a marriage breakup, a serious illness, losing our job – will come along and jolt us out of our carefully managed reality, either out of the blue, or, much more likely, because our unconscious has engineered it.

5. The more you heal, the better you can manifest your true wishes

Toward the end of this book, I talked about the lemniscate, or the infinity symbol (same thing really). The one side of the shape balances the other. I imagine this symbol in constant motion, with one side flowing into the other, around and around. Like a spiral, this represents to me the constant movement of experience, energy in, energy out, inspiration/action of the universe.

In the tarot, the Magician card is always depicted with this symbol present (it also appears on many other cards in the deck). The figure of the Magician, in his traditional image, stands with one hand raised to the heavens and one hand pointing down to the earth. His stance is like a lightning rod, poised for universal energy to flow through him and into whatever project, spell or creation he is focusing on. The Magician accepts the flow of energy in the universe – the healing, if you will – and, with his other hand, makes stuff happen.

When we do our healing work, we start to clear out that big Indiana Jones warehouse of trauma and stuck emotion and old thought patterns in ourselves. As we do so, we make room for new stuff. New relationships, new habits, new patterns.

6. Being honest with yourself about what your true wishes are is hard, but necessary

One of the people who has been most influential on my thoughts regarding healing is Carolyn Elliott,[1] an American occultist-cum-life coach whose phrase "having is evidence of wanting" really resonates with me. Carolyn's theory is that if something exists in our lives, it's because we want it – even if we might not want to admit we want it. Like the idea we talked about earlier, that the unconscious is running the show, having is evidence of wanting really means that not all our deep desires or drivers are "good" or "respectable". Sometimes these patterns are born out of trauma. I'd like to chime in again here and clarify that this **doesn't** mean that when we get cancer or AIDS it's because we really secretly wanted it. This is not what Carolyn's theory is about.

For example, one might always attract relationships with others that are distant, overly critical, or even disrespectful and abusive. If a pattern keeps repeating in this way, it's you that in some way "wants" it in your life, usually because it's familiar – perhaps mimicking an early relationship with a parent who may have been distant, critical or even abusive. It's not your conscious mind seeking out these relationships. Consciously, we all want to be respected and loved. It's the elephant, going for what feels familiar.

---

[1]   I included her book *Existential Kink* in my reading list. Highly recommended.

"Having is evidence of wanting" is a great way to look at your life, look at what is there and isn't there, and conclude some logical truths about what might be in your unconscious from that. If we attract overly critical partners, we might have some old patterning in there somewhere about being unworthy or unconfident. If we constantly find ourselves the victim in different situations, is there a part of us – a part we would rather not acknowledge – that enjoys the attention, the drama and the experience? Is being a victim triggering a wounded child in the unconscious?

Carolyn goes a step further and says that after we've identified what we obviously want on some level, even though it might be distasteful to us, the best way to deal with it is to love it as shamelessly as we can. She advises becoming as turned on as we can about our nasty needs – perhaps our need to control others, or to be controlled in some way, or our desire to please others, or our fears of not being loved, of being ignored, of being bullied. Any of these things and anything else that might be in there.

If we can first become aware of some of the unconscious patterns (bring them into the conscious) and *then* love those things about ourselves without judgement so much that they actually become erotic to us, then that's a radical act of self-acceptance and love. And, ironically, once we have taken such pleasure in the things we might have found shameful (I'm too fat/shy/timid/loud/take up too much space/too stupid/too intelligent/nerdy/etc.), they cease to have the power that they once did. It's the same as what Jung said. *"Until you make the unconscious conscious, it will direct your life and you will call it fate."*

I know, for example, that despite me saying as loudly as I liked in the past that material possessions didn't matter to me, material possessions *are* important to me. I want a good car. I want nice things for my home and when I go away somewhere I like to stay somewhere nice. So what? Nothing wrong with that. But for years I was trying to convince myself, and the world, that I was a as-long-as-you've-got-love-you-can-live-in-a-shoebox-in-the-rain-and-it-doesn't-matter kind of person. No judgement if that's who you are, but I am not. Better to own whoever you are.

I think what I'm trying to say here is that simply by looking at our lives, we can see what programmes we have running in our brains – or indeed, in our energy systems. And if, when you've done that, you decide that *isn't* what you want going forward, then you know what needs to be healed, left behind and moved on from.

7. Healing comes to different people in different ways

What's right for you might not be right for me and vice versa. Horses for courses. My advice is to try different stuff out. If it's not for you, you never have to do it again. But if it is, then go again. Gong baths didn't do it for me, but many people love them. Some people like acupuncture. I haven't tried it but it sounds amazing. Breathwork might not be for everyone (although I recommend it to everyone). Whatever you do, do something.

8. Life is constantly presenting you with opportunities to heal. You just might not like them when they show up

That annoying guy on Twitter? Opportunity to heal. Being in debt? Opportunity to heal. Leaving a relationship? Opportunity to heal. Hating your job? Opportunity to heal. Being ill? Opportunity to heal. Argument with your friend? Opportunity to heal.

None of my examples are pleasant. Life is frequently not pleasant. We all know this. I'm not suggesting that any of my examples are easy to heal from, either. Or that we will always heal, especially from certain illnesses. The point is that we can still come to terms with whatever it is and accept it as part of our life's journey. Acceptance doesn't mean approval. You can still act to change things that you feel are wrong in the world. But there are some things that acceptance it is the ultimate solution to, and a coming-to-terms-with may include protesting against something.

Once you adjust your perception of the world from "If I'm not happy all the time, something is wrong" to "The world is a sophisticated playground specifically made to challenge me, and I love it just as it is in all its disgusting, dark, irritating glory AND its beautiful kindness and love," you're going to be way ahead here, believe me.

Remember the thing about Babalon and loving everything? The dark and the light? If we give ourselves permission to love everything in ourselves – even the bits that until now we were ashamed of or disliked about ourself – then we will find it much easier to love and accept everything "outside" us (I say "outside" because really there is no inside and outside; it's an illusion. Recognizing the connectedness of everything is terrifying, though, because that also means we all have responsibility for everything, which is why we continue to believe in dualities like inside/outside, light/dark, masculine/feminine. It makes it way easier for us to function).

Like Tiffany taught me in lockdown, being grateful for everything is powerful because it's like a supercharged acceptance. Not only are you accepting of everything, you are actively grateful for it. You LOVE everything. And when you're operating at loving everything, everything is possible.

Like Matthew said when I interviewed him, how we behave with other people reflects how we feel about ourselves. If we are constantly in a state of self-judgement, self-hate, if we have low self-esteem, if we cannot love the one person who creates our reality – the only truth we can ever really be sure of – then what does it say about our ability to accept and love others? But if we give ourselves a break and listen to our hearts, listen to our wounded inner children and give ourselves the healing we need, whatever it is, without judgement, that is an act of love.

9. Accept life how it is and love it how it is

Tiffany, my psychic healer friend, taught me this. Gratefulness will set you free. It genuinely works. Again, gratefulness does not mean you don't also want something better in your life; it's a state of mind that, ironically, makes it easier for the 'even better' bits to materialize because you are not forming negative attachments to certain things (i.e. passionately hating and resenting them).

10. Having "everything" is not the goal

This was a big realization for me.

Overcoming a kind of continual dissatisfaction with what I have and the perception of who I am (note: the perception of who I am, rather than who I really am, which is a changeable concept as it is for all of us) has been a lifelong struggle for me.

Despite what I may have wanted to admit about myself in the past, I care about material possessions and financial security. I CARE. I love expensive, top-quality clothes and home furnishings and I totally understand the need for a top-of-the-range kettle.

I get a peaceful feeling from the bills being paid and everything working harmoniously in the house. I am stressed out by leaks and dirty floors and half-finished DIY tasks. I love high-quality home décor and could pass a blindfold test with budget and luxury brand food any day of the week.

For a long time, I was sort of ashamed of this part of me. But now, here I am, having accepted it and loved it and – know what? It works for me. It might not be you, but that's okay. You have your thing.

I tried to believe that I didn't care about money for most of my life. I grew up not having any, with the philosophy that money doesn't matter. For me, that turned into a deep aversion to having it at all, and, as I've talked about earlier, I spent most of my adult life trying to get rid of it as quickly as humanly possible until I hit a debt wall and had to face up to money as an entity; I had to admit that it DOES matter, I DO care about it and, until humanity evolves a system of living that no longer needs it, then I had to have it too.

HOWEVER, do I need to be a billionaire? No. I do not need to have EVERYTHING.

I subscribe to *Vogue* every month (subscribing = cheaper than buying it off the shelf every month – look at me making responsible choices!) because I love fashion and pretty dresses. But, for many years, I banned myself from reading *Vogue* because it always made me very sad and dissatisfied with my own life. Why wasn't I jetting off to Sardinia on a private jet? Why didn't I own Missoni homewares? Why wasn't I at Paris Fashion Week? This was genuinely my internal monologue of woe reading it. Pathetic, right?

I didn't read *Vogue* for years. How sad (and intensely privileged) is that? A fashion magazine had so much power over me that I literally couldn't pick it up for fear of my world crashing around me (from an emotional point of view). That *want* was intense; that shadow of the poverty consciousness I had as a child and into adulthood stayed with me and ran the show for a long time. It wasn't just wealth; it was success too. Why hadn't I written an international bestseller? Why hadn't I won the Booker Prize? I was holding myself up to ridiculous standards for reasons I didn't even understand.

The place I have come to, though, is that EVERYTHING – which for me equated to a billionaire lifestyle, and international acclaim – was not the goal. In fact, both of those things are ridiculous things to want. No, really! They are. Think about it. Billions are more than you as an individual need (I mean, I'm fine with MILLIONS. A million pounds nowadays is not what it was) unless you're funding a large public health programme – in which case, good luck to you and off you go.

And winning a literary prize, well, having seen many a literary prize from behind the scenes now, I can tell you that they are very nice to have, as is the prize money if there is any, but they are ABSOLUTELY NO REFLECTION on whether your book is worthy or necessary in any way, or anything more than the best of a small selection of books that some other people liked. All that judgement is, is ultimately a small group of people with certain opinions and biases sitting in a room and coming to an agreement based on a set of niche requirements; it's completely subjective AND often very dependent on one or two loud voices in the room. Is it that important? Does it validate the person who wrote the book in a deeply profound way? Is it the prime motivation for creating a work of art? Not really.

Why did I want to win a significant literary prize? Ego. I wanted to be feted as one of the great minds of her generation. I wanted people to admire me. I wanted to be interviewed by the broadsheets as a Clever Person. Really, when you boil all of that down, it comes to what humans always want, which is to be loved, and to be seen.

I didn't ever actually have any need to receive praise specifically for my work, just like I never needed my teachers' or my parents' praise for my work as a child. I just did it because I wanted to, and I knew it was good. So, my fantasy goal of being a well-known Clever Clogs wasn't about being recognized for my work. When I really get down to it, recognition is nice, but it doesn't drive me – I am a "the work is its own reward" sort of person. What was driving this goal – and its related sense of disappointment in Self because it hadn't happened – was that inner child desperately wanting love and attention.

You can also tell that this was/is an inner child desire, also, because it's a variant of the "wanting to be a pop star" or "wanting to marry Michael J Fox" (one of my earliest fantasies) ideas we often have as children. It's not an adult goal, like having good health, having great friends or a fulfilling life/work balance.

Also, I don't actually want to be known as a newspaper Clever Person Who Is Asked To Comment on Things because a) there are many far cleverer people than me out there – I mean, my memory for facts is absolutely terrible, for one thing, and if interviewed there's no way I could be as succinct as the people who actually are Clever People Who Are Asked To Comment on Things; b) I love anonymity and would hate being a celebrity of any kind and have everyone knowing my business; and c) it's actually just not that interesting. To me, anyway.

Having "everything" is not the goal. Once you set those parameters aside – the goals that, in my case, my fears set for me – what are you left with?

Sadly, it's the naff answer you suspected all along. It's being happy with what you have, in the present. Today, I'm sitting near to the window on a November day looking at the yellow leaves of a tree against the bright blue sky while tapping away on my laptop. My cat is lying next to me, doing fishy yawns (yuck) and I've got half an eye on the clock, wondering about what I'm having for lunch. And this is a perfect moment. I am not hungry or thirsty or exhausted or in pain; I have a house I live in and peace and quiet and a robin hopping among the fallen leaves outside and this is my goal. Not those individual things, but a state of peace and detachment from wanting things or believing that my life would be better if I only had something else or was someone else. I am lucky to have what I have. I have also worked very hard to have my life and I am very, very grateful for it.

11. You can always have a biscuit and a cup of tea

Yes! You can! What a relief. Let's have one now! I think we all deserve it.

We looked at having a custard cream on the cover for the book, but the designer came up with the spiral shaped lolly[2] instead, and I think we can all agree it looks a bit more exciting.

But, you know, I have consumed a heck of a lot of biscuits (or "cookies" for my American readers who may have been thinking about THEIR type of biscuit all the way through this book and been thoroughly confused) on my healing journey, and I don't plan on stopping any time soon. Life's too short.

That's it, really. Life *is* very short. We cram a lot in to our time here: education, family, friends, work, love, heartbreak, illness, death. Regardless of what we do and what we heal and don't heal, who we love and don't love, or whether we become billionaire Booker Prize-winning egomaniacs, one day, it's all over and what's done is done.

---

[2] See what we did there?

Who knows what happens after? Some people claim they do. We all have our beliefs. Perhaps all our time in this challenging hell hole/paradise[3] of a world accounts for nothing and there's no point in healing anything. You die anyway, right? (I feel like I deserve a biscuit for this clever segue from biscuits to death.)

Maybe. But I'm thinking that if you're reading this, you probably don't think that.

I don't believe that.

I don't claim to have any more answers than anyone else, and all I really have is my own experience. But to me it makes sense not to value our experiences or what we learn as a good or bad thing, but to accept them all, warts n' all, and in so doing learn something about ourselves and about life.

Maybe Earth is a place where souls are given bodies and come to live in the material realm for a while. Maybe this place is a school, like a nursery, where we get dropped off for a while to learn our human lessons. And healing is a part of that.

Maybe humans are hosts for bacteria and it's them that are running the show. Maybe all life forms think they're running things and going through evolutionary peaks and troughs. It's not going so well for the bees right now, if so.

Maybe we are part of the universe dreaming itself, and our healing journeys are part of that gloriously intertextual dream, made of quadrillions of connections and sparks of light and stars and souls. Maybe the religions – or the spiritual systems – are right. God is Love. We are Love.

Whatever the great answer to everything is, healing seems to me to be part of the modus operandi of being a human on Earth. This place does nothing but challenge us and give us countless opportunities for experience, whether that be to experience emotions, the physical world – Food! Sex! Cushions! Exercise! – thought and cognition or drive and determinism.

If anything, healing our emotions gives us more opportunity to take in everything the world has to offer, and to be freer to

---

3   Delete as appropriate.

bend the malleable shape of existence into a life that bears the closest resemblance to whatever is our true will – or our mission in life – is. Or, even more likely: when we have integrated and dissolved our trauma, we are able to realign naturally to our true purpose, like a washing line caught in a tree which is released and snapped back into place. Thinking about it like this, there's actually no work to be done in bending the world to your will after having let go of what was holding you back. After a certain point, you are just operating at the level of what Aleister Crowley would call True Will, or what my reiki teachers called Highest Will.

Emotional healing also gives us the opportunity to do the most shocking and terrifying thing of all: love. Love ourselves, just as we are; love others just as they are, and love this world in all its terrible glory.

Well, on that bombshell, I think it's time to stop harping on about life and maybe live it a little.

Pass the biscuit tin. I'll put the kettle on.

RECOMMENDED READING

I've recommended and mentioned a lot of books as I rambled along, so here they are as a reminder. I've also added in others that I haven't mentioned that are good. I've also arranged them under subject headings because I'm nice like that.

Witchcraft

Witchcraft is such a varied practice that I could write pages of recommendations for all the different takes, traditions and cultures within it. The best thing to do is go and have a browse in your nearest esoteric bookshop and see what speaks to you – or ask someone in the shop what they'd recommend. These are some of the books I've either mentioned already or ones I rate myself.

Auryn, Mat, *Psychic Witch*, Llewellyn, 2020
Elliott, Carolyn, *Existential Kink*, Red Wheel/Weiser, 2020
Farrar, Janet and Stewart Ferrar, *A Witch's Bible*, The Crowood Press, 2002
Frater U D, *Practical Sigil Magic*, Llewellyn, 2012
Gary, Gemma, *The Black Toad*, Troy Books, 2019
Grey, Peter, *The Red Goddess*, Scarlet Imprint, 2016
Grossman, Pam, *Waking the Witch*, Gallery Books, 2019

Morgan, Levannah, *A Witch's Mirror,* Capall Bann Publishing, 2021

Rankine, David and Sorite Rankine, *The Guises of The Morrigan*, Avalonia Press, 2012

Vincent, Mark, *The Sigil Secret*, Palaysia Publishers, 2021

Wachter, Adrian, *Six Ways: Approaches and Entries for Practical Magic*, Red Temple Press, 2018

Wachter, Adrian, *Weaving Fate*, Red Temple Press, 2020

West, Kate, *A Real Witch's Handbook,* Thorsons, 2016

Woodfield, Stephanie, *Celtic Lore & Spellcraft of the Dark Goddess,* Llewellyn, 2011

Reiki/energy healing

Brennan, Barbara Ann, *Light Emerging*, illustrated by Thomas J Schneider & Joan Tartaglia, Bantam Books, 2011

Brennan, Barbara Ann & Smith, Jos A, *Hands of Light*, Bantam Books, 2011

Lübeck, Walter & Petter, Frank Arjava, *The Spirit of Reiki,* Lotus Press, 2001

Shamanism

Harner, Michael, *The Way of the Shaman*, Harper San Francisco, 1992

Ingerman, Sandra, *Shamanic Journeying: A Beginner's Guide,* Sounds True, Inc. 2008 (this comes with a CD of drumming tracks to listen to for journeying, but I've also found them online free on YouTube)

Ingerman, Sandra, *Soul Retrieval*, HarperOne, 2010

Some, Malidoma Patrice, *Of Water and the Spirit*, Penguin, 1995

Sex
Carellas, Barbara & Sprinkle, Dr Annie, *Urban Tantra*, Ten Speed Press, 2017
Richardson, Diana, *The Heart of Tantric Sex*, O Books, 2003
Pailet, Xanet, *Living an Orgasmic Life*, Mango Press, 2018

Sound healing
Gaynor, Mitchell L, M.D., *The Healing Power of Sound*, Shambhala Publications, 2002
McKusick, Eileen Day, *Tuning the Human Biofield*, Healing Arts Press, 2021

General healing
Farmer, Dr Steven D, *Healing Ancestral Karma*, Hierophant Publishing, 2014
Fleche, Christian, *The Biogenealogy Sourcebook*, Healing Arts Press, 2008
Obissier, Patrick, *Biogenealogy*, Healing Arts Press, 2005
Virtue, Doreen, PhD, *Archangels and Ascended Masters,* Hay House, 2004
Wardle, Tiffany, *Learn Lemurian Healing*, Vintage Wisdom, 2013

Inspiring memoirs about healing and grief
Bell, Poorna, *Stronger: Changing Everything I Knew About Women's Strength*, Bluebird, 2021
Cho, Catherine, *Inferno: A Memoir of Motherhood and Madness*, Bloomsbury, 2021
Coles, Reverend Richard, *The Madness of Grief*, Weidenfeld & Nicholson, 2021
Dockrill, Laura, *What Have I Done? Motherhood, Mental Illness & Me*, Vintage, 2021
Rentzenbrink, Cathy, *A Manual for Heartbreak*, Picador, 2017

Winfrey, Oprah & Perry, Dr Bruce, *What Happened To You? Conversations on Trauma, Resilience and Healing*, Bluebird, 2021

Other books of interest
Kahneman, Daniel, *Thinking, Fast and Slow*, Penguin, 2012
Perez, Caroline Criado, *Invisible Women*, Vintage, 2020

Instagram accounts of interest
The Holistic Psychologist, Dr Nicole LePera:
@the.holistic.psychologist
Marie is a Trauma Informed Grief and end-of-life doula who works with people to rebuild their lives around loss. You can also find her at www.empoweredthroughgrief.com and on Instagram @empowered_through_grief

The Menopause Doctor, Dr Louise Newson:
@menopause_doctor
Louise is a GP and menopause specialist, founder of @themenocharity and the @balancemenopause app.

The Ladybird Purse:
@ladybirdpurse
Keris Stainton writes a newsletter about women, midlife and money which you can subscribe to at theladybirdpurse. substack.com

Somatic Experiencing International:
@somaticexperiencingint
A non-profit organisation dedicated to transforming lives through healing, based on the teachings of Dr Peter A Levine.

Healing from PTSD:
@healingfromptsd
This is a personal account from Madeline Popelka in which she shares her experience of PTSD and her wisdom gained from it. She's also a writer and mental health advocate and you can find out more about her on www.madelinepopelka.com

Unapologetically Surviving:
@unapologeticallysurviving
A community of trauma survivors, supporters and allies promoting healing, resilience and empowerment.

Healing + Complex-PTSD:
@healing.and.cptsd
Community for complex trauma survivors. You can also find them at www.healingandcptsd.com

Interviewees

Tiffany Wardle: www.tiffanywardle.com and on Instagram @tiffanywardleofficial
Ana Isabel: Ana mentions the Michael Newton Institute which you can find at www.newtoninstitute.org. You can find Ana on www.lifeastrologer.com and www.lifehypnosis.net for astrology, past life regression and hypnotherapy or on Instagram @lifeastrologer and @lifehypnosis
Laura Daligan: www.lauradaligan.com and on Instagram @lauraredwitch
Maria Wilson: www.mariawilson.co.uk
Matthew Donnachie: www.innerbalancelife.co.uk

I did my reiki one and two with an organization called **Acorn To Oak**, who also offer breathwork and other therapies, and whom I would recommend wholeheartedly. You can find them at www.acorntooak.co.uk

ACKNOWLEDGEMENTS

Thank you to Marco Visconti for his wisdom about Babalon, and to all my incredibly wise interviewees. Thank you to all the therapists and magical folk I have met along the way of my own healing journey, all of them too many to list here – I have learnt from all of you.

Thank you to my parents, my best teachers, and to Ella Chappell and Sophie Elletson for being wonderful editors. Thanks also to Melinda Salisbury for being kind enough to connect me with Ella in the first place, and to all the kind booksellers that will stock this book.

Last, thank you to my family.

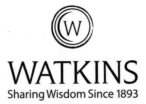

WATKINS

Sharing Wisdom Since 1893

The story of Watkins began in 1893, when scholar of esotericism John Watkins founded our bookshop, inspired by the lament of his friend and teacher Madame Blavatsky that there was nowhere in London to buy books on mysticism, occultism or metaphysics. That moment marked the birth of Watkins, soon to become the publisher of many of the leading lights of spiritual literature, including Carl Jung, Rudolf Steiner, Alice Bailey and Chögyam Trungpa.

Today, the passion at Watkins Publishing for vigorous questioning is still resolute. Our stimulating and groundbreaking list ranges from ancient traditions and complementary medicine to the latest ideas about personal development, holistic wellbeing and consciousness exploration. We remain at the cutting edge, committed to publishing books that change lives.

DISCOVER MORE AT:
www.watkinspublishing.com

Read our blog

Watch and listen to
our authors in action

Sign up to
our mailing list

We celebrate conscious, passionate, wise and happy living.
Be part of that community by visiting

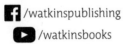 /watkinspublishing   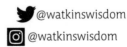 @watkinswisdom

/watkinsbooks   @watkinswisdom